The Healing
Power of
tea

About the Author

Caroline Dow (Boulder, CO) has been a tea leaf reader and aromatherapist for thirty years and conducts popular workshops on tea leaf reading around the US and abroad. Author of sixteen books under various pen names, she also owns and manages an online aromatherapy company. She holds a PhD in Luso-Brazilian Studies and received a Fulbright Dissertation Research Fellowship to Brazil. Her book *Magic from Brazil: Recipes, Spells and Rituals* (Llewellyn, 2001) chronicles those experiences. Three books she has written for Llewellyn have won national and state awards: *Complete Book of the Psychic Arts* (2000), *Fuego Angelical* (2000), and *Tea Leaf Reading for Beginners* (2011).

To Write the Author

If you wish to contact the author or would like more information about this book, please write to the author in care of Llewellyn Worldwide, and we will forward your request. Both the author and publisher appreciate hearing from you and learning of your enjoyment of this book and how it has helped you. Llewellyn Worldwide cannot guarantee that every letter written to the author can be answered, but all will be forwarded. Please write to:

Caroline Dow
℅ Llewellyn Worldwide
2143 Wooddale Drive
Woodbury, MN 55125-2989

Please enclose a self-addressed stamped envelope for reply,
or $1.00 to cover costs. If outside the USA, enclose
an international postal reply coupon.

CAROLINE DOW

The Healing Power *of* tea

**Simple Teas & Tisanes
to Remedy and Rejuvenate
Your Health**

Llewellyn Publications
Woodbury, Minnesota

FIRST EDITION
Second Printing, 2014

Book design by Bob Gaul
Cover design by Ellen Lawson
Cover image by Ellen Lawson
Editing by Laura Graves

Llewellyn Publications is a registered trademark of Llewellyn Worldwide Ltd.

Library of Congress Cataloging-in-Publication Data
Dow, Caroline.
  The healing power of tea: simple teas & tisanes to remedy and rejuvenate your health/Caroline Dow.—First edition.
     pages cm
  Includes bibliographical references.
  ISBN 978-0-7387-4033-1
1. Tea—Therapeutic use. 2. Tea—Health aspects. I. Title.
  RM251.D69 2014
  615.3'21—dc23
                                        2014026213

Llewellyn Publications
A Division of Llewellyn Worldwide Ltd.
2143 Wooddale Drive
Woodbury, MN 55125-2989
www.llewellyn.com

Printed in the United States of America

Contents

Acknowledgments

Acknowledgments go to acquisitions editor Amy Glaser and the vision committee, whose many comments and suggestions helped shape this book into its final form.

Introduction

This book is about how tea and herbal infusions can help heal the body. It also details ways to drink tea and herbal teas as a preventative measure. The text focuses specifically on the therapeutic value of tea and herbal teas. Included is updated data about kinds of tea and their health benefits, and descriptions of grades and popular types. Ailments and teas to help alleviate them are highlighted. Information about blending, preparation, consumption, and how to prepare herbal infusions for healthy living is also covered. Gardening tips are offered for those inclined to grow their own herbs for tea making. The appendix includes suggested recipes. A glossary of tea terms as well as reference data for the scientific studies quoted are provided at the end of the book.

The book is a manual for those who wish to learn more about the healing power of tea for healthy living. Unfortunately, neither tea nor herbal teas are a cure-all for any ailment—they are supplemental drinks to be consumed for better health and enjoyment. They can be ingested when standard medications engender too many side effects. Unlike standard medicine, which is strong and meant to root out disease, teas and other botanical preparations exert gentle effects on the body. They stimulate a person's natural defenses against disease, and thus work best as a preventative or for minor or chronic conditions such as a cold, headache, or indigestion.

Therefore, the information presented is not meant to be a substitute for professional medical care. It is offered as a guide to those who wish to engage in additional alternative treatments. If you are suffering from any ailment whatsoever, it is strongly suggested you see a qualified, licensed medical professional.

One

About Tea

This chapter relates a brief history of tea on how it has been used for healing and healthy living. The chapter goes on to describe what tea is, different grades and types of tea, some health benefits of drinking tea, and current tea trends.

The Sumerians were the first people to supply a record of the medicinal properties of botanicals, which they engraved on clay tablets around 3000 BCE. However, the Chinese were the first to discover the tea botanical. They called this substance "The River of Jade" because, at first, they drank only unprocessed green leaves. They valued tea so much for its health benefits that they likened this drink to the precious mineral jade. In 780 CE, *Ch'a Ching, The*

Classic of Tea, was the first book written on the history, medicinal properties, and cultivation of tea. In it, the author states the health benefits the Chinese people believed were derived from tea. These benefits included longevity, cures for headache and nervousness, and the ability to keep a person alert.

In 1191 CE, the founder of Zen Buddhism brought the first tea seeds from China to Japan. This monk planted the seeds at his monastery in Kyoto. As far as healthy living is concerned, both Chinese and Japanese monks mostly drank tea to stay alert during meditation. During the Chinese Ming Dynasty (1368–1644), modern methods of steeping green, oolong, and black leaves in teapots and cups were developed. Now most people in these countries drink tea for pleasure as well as for healthy living.

Tea was introduced to Europeans by the Dutch in 1610 via a shipment of green tea from Japan. The Dutch touted the drink for its ability to cure headaches, keep a person alert, and to promote longevity, just as the Chinese had done. Catherine of Braganza, the Portuguese queen to Charles II of England, was already drinking tea in Portugal before she married, and she introduced the beverage to the British as a healthy alternative to alcohol. She too believed that tea cured headaches, kept a person alert, and promoted longevity. Eventually tea consumption spread throughout the world. Today people drink it because they like the taste and also because they believe in tea's ability to cure a variety of ills, including heart disease, digestive problems, headaches, diseases of the immune system, respiratory system, nervous system, and more. These ailments and tea's alleged ability to help keep a person alert, promote longevity, and alleviate symptoms of disease are detailed later in this chapter and throughout the book.

There are many drinks, including herbal concoctions, which people generally refer to as "tea." People involved in the tea industry maintain that all *real* tea—meaning black, oolong, green, yellow, and white—comes from the same plant, a kind of camellia (*Camellia sinensis* and *Thea sinensis*). This flowering evergreen grows in the wild as a tree. Growers prune it back to shrub height to make harvesting the leaves easier. The tea bush thrives at high altitudes in humid climates near the equator. It grows best when the leaves are shaded from the searing sun. In fact, one varietal, Gyokuro, is cultivated completely in shade.

Bushes are grown on plantations known as tea gardens. One or more gardens tended under a single management are called a "tea estate." Teas from different regions are often blended together. For example, English Breakfast Tea includes teas from China, India, and Sri Lanka. If a blend comes entirely from teas grown on the same estate, it is called a Single Estate Tea and is often relatively expensive.

Although tea originated in China, currently only around 10 percent of the production for international markets is cultivated there. These days India, Japan, and Sri Lanka are major producers. Tea is also harvested in such far-flung locations as Australia, Argentina, Kenya,

Korea, Mozambique, Vietnam, Indonesia, Chile, Papua/ New Guinea, Guatemala, and Zaire. Tea has even been produced since colonial times in the US. It continues to be harvested, albeit in small amounts, in South Carolina, Alabama, Hawaii, and Washington state.

Teas are sold in different grades. The grade of a tea has little to do with the health benefits to be derived from the tea and therefore falls outside the purview of this book. But it should be noted that the grade of a tea does affect taste. Grading tea is a complicated business, and different types are assessed differently. For example, black teas are classified according to leaf size and appearance. Whether the leaf is whole or broken makes little difference. Oolongs, on the other hand, are whole leaf teas, judged according to leaf quality and taste.

Before launching into a discussion of the health benefits of tea, it is a good idea to describe what kinds of tea are being mentioned. Five different types of tea all come from the same bush. Their health benefits are more or less the same because all tea comes from the one plant. Due to different processing techniques, there are slight differences in the health benefits of each type, which also makes them taste different, so you may choose one type over the other according to personal preference. One significant difference between types of tea is the amount of caffeine each contains. This is the result of different processing techniques, chiefly the length of time the tea leaves are allowed to ferment before drying. This fermentation process, known as oxidation, occurs after the leaves are left to dry on racks. Then they are twisted and rolled to break up the leaf cells and release the essential oils, which remain on the leaves.

Following are short descriptions of the five types of tea along with some of their health benefits as well as a general description of herbal teas. Taste is mentioned because the only real differences between the five types of tea that come from the *Camellia sinensis* bush are their flavors.

White Tea

These delicate teas are produced on a very limited scale. In order to harvest white tea, the buds are picked before they open, along with the youngest leaves. This meticulous harvest is allowed to wilt very slightly and then is dried using hot air to prevent oxidation. This process creates a smooth-tasting, pale green to clear liquor that emits a delicate grassy aroma. According to a study written up in the medical journal *Nutrition and Cancer* by G. Santana-Rios, G. A. Orner, M. Xu, M. Izquierdo-Pulido, and R. H. Dashwood, white tea, along with the other types of tea, is thought to stimulate the nerve cells of the brain and reduce occurrences of cancers of the stomach, colon, rectum, bladder, and prostate by attacking free radicals that can accumulate in the tissues.

Yellow Tea

Yellow tea is a type of green tea. Yellow teas are produced in very limited quantities and only in China. In fact, the quantities are so limited that this tea is difficult to obtain in the US. Because this tea oxidizes more slowly than green teas, the damp leaves turn yellow. The leaves are hand-rolled in cowhide while still damp and then air-dried for a day or more. The health benefits are the same as for white or green teas, but the aroma is flowery and the taste subtle and sweet, without the grassiness associated with most green teas. According to a study performed by N. T. Zaveri in the medical journal *Life Sciences* having to do with tea's medicinal uses in cancer and noncancer applications, yellow tea, as with the other types of tea, can be drunk to prevent and mitigate swelling and inflammation.

Green Tea

Green tea begins its journey to the cup by plucking the top two leaves and unopened leaf buds, the most tender and desirable parts of the tea bush. Harvesting can be accomplished by machine, but truly outstanding green teas are hand-plucked. The leaves are steamed or pan-fired to wither them slightly. Then they are quickly rolled or shaken either by hand or machine to release essential oils and then dried to prevent as much oxidation as possible. This process endows the leaves with a subtle aroma and light grassy taste, signature characteristics of many green teas.

All types of tea facilitate weight loss, but green tea is thought to be especially good at helping a person shed extra pounds. This is because as with all five types of tea, green tea increases fat oxidation by thermogenesis (heat production) in the human body. It also lowers LDL cholesterol levels, which makes it a good choice for diabetics. Many studies conducted over the years have shown that green tea prevents diabetes, but one study performed at the University of Shizuoka, Japan by Yoko Fukino claims that green tea can control blood sugar levels that are already very high.

Oolong Tea

Oolongs are mainly made in China and Taiwan. They come in a variety of flavors, aromas, and colors. Unlike green and white teas, oolong teas can be infused several times. The term *oolong* is a variation of a word in Chinese that means "black dragon." This type of tea originated in the Fujian province of China. Oolong teas are partially oxidized teas. To create an oolong, leaves are withered and gently shaken to bruise the edges, then semi-oxidized, rolled, and dried. The process results in a tea that displays a wide range of flavors. The antioxidants in oolong tea, as well as in other types, fight infectious diseases and detoxifies the liver. According to a study in the *Journal of Medicinal Food,* this type of tea as well as green tea can mitigate certain symptoms of

Parkinson's disease such as reduced memory and lack of focus.

Black Tea

Black tea is probably the type most familiar to readers. It is served frequently in restaurants and until the recent upsurge of interest in this beverage, was almost the only kind found on grocery store shelves. The leaves are withered and either rolled or cut. The key difference between black teas and all other kinds is that the leaves are fully oxidized before being dried or fired.

When it comes to nutrition, robust black tea is associated with good health and energy. This is because it contains more caffeine than other types of tea. It is also the reason black teas tend to be more flavorful than other types. Black tea as well as the other types of tea may decrease LDL cholesterol levels, increase the ability of blood vessels to respond to stress, and thus reduce the risk for hardening of the arteries, heart attack, and stroke. This claim has been made in a study performed by V. E. Steele, G. J. Kelloff, D. Balentine, et al. in the medical journal *Carcinogenesis*.

Herbal Teas

The term "herbal tea" is a misnomer. There is no such thing as an herbal tea. Terms such as "red tea" or "rooibos tea" for example, are not true teas. Those beverages come from a totally different bush. Drinks made from botanicals other than the *Camellia sinensis* bush should be called herbal infusions or tisanes. However, since this book is directed to the general public and most laypeople refer to herbal infusions as herbal teas, this book also will use the term "herbal tea" to describe these beverages.

Herbal teas can be concocted from a single botanical or combinations of botanicals. They can be brewed from flowers, leaves, stems, seeds, and even roots. Herbal teas have similar health benefits to true teas. They may even contain more because they are harvested from a variety of plants which have different characteristics.

As to healthy living, herbal teas are consumed in the same way as tea is drunk to benefit the brain, ears, mouth, skin, lungs, esophagus, liver, breasts, bones, joints, digestive system, immune system, cardiovascular system, and to maintain a healthy weight. Chapter 6 provides a list of ailments and herbal botanicals other than tea used to treat them.

Although this book concentrates on the nutritional and medicinal benefits of tea, this does not mean you cannot also take pleasure in drinking tea as people all over the world have done for millennia. While tea is as old as the Himalayas, contemporary society has only recently reembraced the joys of taking tea. And as things usually go in our consumer-oriented society, this rediscovery has led to several new products as well as traditional products repackaged and marketed for contemporary times. Following are some trends.

Artisan Teas
(also called Artistic or Artisanal Teas)

Premium full-leaf teas, sometimes called "connoisseur's teas" or "collectors' teas," consist of black, green, oolong, or white teas sewn into blossoms or rosettes. They are handcrafted in small batches, sometimes blended for a special occasion, an individual, or even at a particular time of day, season, or year. Artisan teas used to be rare, but are gaining in popularity in spite of their high price tag. To brew an artisan tea, place a blossom in the bottom of a cup and pour boiling water over it. Watch while the rosette "blooms" into a pretty peony or anemone flower. As with all teas, artisan teas are drunk to protect the body from the profusion of free radicals, mitigate clogging of the arteries, and fight various cancers.

Bubble Tea

Also known as boba or pearl tea, this beverage was invented at a tea kiosk outside a school in Taiwan during the early 1980s. Tea vendors would set up stands in the street and vie for business as thirsty children left for home in the hot afternoon. To gain a leg up on the competition, one concessioner decided to add sweet flavoring to cold, infused tea and shake it until it formed bubbles. The intriguing drink caught on immediately. Around the same time, a Taiwanese man named Liu Han-Chieh began adding chewy tapioca pearls to his tea in a successful effort to appeal to children.

Pearls can be black, white, or transparent in color. The drink is served in a clear glass so the consumer can view the pretty pearls on the bottom. Tapioca pearls are marble-size, so you need a fat straw to suck them up. Sometimes fresh fruit, milk, and/or crushed ice are added to make a bubble tea milkshake. This drink is a far cry from traditional tea, but it does represent an enduring tea-based trend. As to its health benefits, other than those stated above that apply to all teas, the fresh fruit and milk add vitamin and mineral content and the sugar adds carbohydrates, which transforms into energy in the body.

Chai Tea

This fragrant blend, also called masala chai, hails from India, where it is a tradition deep-rooted in the culture. The drink features black or green tea brewed with milk, sugar, and spices. You can find chai as a dry blend, in tea-bag form or even ready to drink at the grocery, and nowadays it is served at most coffeehouses. If you make your chai from green tea, you will reap green tea's health benefits along with the calcium and vitamin D found in milk. Then there are the spices. Besides tasting good, cardamom, cinnamon, cloves, coriander, cumin, ginger, nutmeg, and pepper—some or all of which are included in the mix— are healthy and nutritious. For example, cinnamon is an antiseptic, antifungal, and astringent. When a woman is about to give birth, clove will strengthen uterine contractions and help ease delivery. Ginger is beneficial for flatulent colic, diarrhea, kidney trouble, and chest complaints.

Chocolate Tea

Combining tea with chocolate is another hot trend. Chocolate is the product of cacao seeds, commonly called beans. Purplish-pink beans grow on stalks inside the fruit of a 40-foot evergreen native to Mexico, Central, and South America. Embedded in the pulp is the source of what the Aztecs called "food of the gods."

Like tea, cacao beans are harvested, fermented in order to develop more flavor, and then dried. After that, they are cleaned, roasted, and the shells removed. The roasted beans are ground into a liquefied cocoa mass and separated into cocoa butter and fat-free cocoa solids.

Maya, Aztec, and earlier Mesoamerican people believed that each sip of the steaming brew conferred wisdom and knowledge. They also considered chocolate an aphrodisiac. Modern-day scientists have verified the Aztecs' claims by showing that cacao contains the chemical phenyl ethylamine (PEA), which causes the brain to think it is falling in love.

Chocolate is said to have a soothing effect on troubled minds. It combats fatigue and is a quick energizer. A person can walk 150 paces on only one chocolate chip's worth of energy. This substance is rich in potassium and can treat high blood pressure, mild headache, and constipation (when mixed with cayenne). As to its caffeine content, compared to coffee and tea, chocolate is pretty much a lightweight. According to the USDA's National Nutrient Database, three heaping teaspoons of chocolate powder mix renders only 8 mg of caffeine and one envelope of hot chocolate mix will only give you 5 mg. These particular statistics have been chosen to illustrate chocolate's caffeine content because they are the way in which you will most likely mix your chocolate into tea. More information on caffeine and tea is given in succeeding chapters of this book.

As with the addition of milk to tea, the French were the first to think of combining chocolate with tea. In the mid-nineteenth century, the Mariage Frères brothers took over their father's tea importation business. Soon they began blending their own teas and came up with the idea for what would become a famous blend, *Chocolat des Mandarins*—a combination of hot chocolate and black tea. The brothers went on to invent more than two hundred blends.

Besides combining the notable health benefits of both substances, the full-bodied flavor of the tea brightens the chocolate notes.

Fair Trade Teas

The concept of fair trade products was first envisioned in 1988 with the goal to help disadvantaged farmers and artisans in developing countries. For a product to be certified as fair trade, the farmer must adhere to stringent social and environmental controls. Producers also have to establish a just price for their product and guarantee workers a reasonable living wage. The health benefits of fair trade teas are exactly the same as those of other teas. The only reason to buy them instead of standard teas is to help out disadvantaged farmers and artisans in developing nations.

Functional Teas

These designer teas are similar to sports drinks and enhanced waters, except tea is used as a base. Marketed as "healthy drinks," functional teas are supposed to help the consumer keep physically fit, increase physical stamina, manage stress and weight, and boost nutrition. The teas often are sold ready-to-drink for convenience and may be enhanced with vitamins and minerals. It is the tea itself that provides the antioxidants inherent in tea along with the added vitamins and minerals. As far as healthy living is concerned, functional teas are no better or worse than the other types of teas. You could down a cup of white, yellow, green, oolong, or black tea with a multivitamin and produce the same result. You can buy functional teas in the organic section of your supermarket, at organic groceries such as Whole Foods, and at specialty tea shops.

Puerh Tea

Puerh (also spelled "pu-erh" and "puer") is one of the hottest teas on the market today. This large-leaf tea is harvested from ancient trees in the southern mountains of Yunnan province in China. The leaves are truly fermented in mounds rather than oxidized, fired and aged underground while still moist for three months and, in some cases, up to years. To the untrained eye, this process may look a bit like a rotting compost heap. The fermentation process is constantly monitored for temperature and moisture. The end-product is a mellow, earthy flavor, highly regarded by connoisseurs. Although you can order Puerh teas by the cup or pot in most tearooms, it is sold in cakes that require a special pick for removing what is brewed.

The main health benefits associated with puerh tea (other than those inherent in all teas) lie in the Chinese practice of drinking it as a blood purifier and diges-tive aid, especially after a heavy meal. Some swear that puerh makes the ultimate hangover preventative and cure. Popular varieties include the signature black puerh, which has a strong, dark flavor reminiscent of a wet forest floor. For a lighter brew, try green puerh. It begins with a green tea base, and although it eventually turns dark, the green tea flavor modifies the muddy overtones. Another fairly smooth-tasting brew is Puerh Imperial. Tea experts maintain that a fine starter puerh is the one scented with chrysanthemum blossoms. The delicate sweetness of the bloom counterbalances the earthy puerh tones. To accus-tom your palate to puerh tea, it is suggested you try pair-ing it with foods such as chicken, meat, and stir fry.

RTD Teas

RTD simply means "ready to drink." These drinks, usually packaged in plastic bottles or cans, have taken the market by storm because consumers like the convenience and variety of tastes. A small sampling from major chain grocery stores reveals that you can buy black, green, or white tea with or without lemon, diet-sweetened, sweetened with ginseng and honey, or peach and raspberry. Most of these teas contain sugar, so the drinker gets the benefit of added energy that carbohydrates provide. The health benefits of RTD teas are similar to other teas as they all originate in the same bush. General benefits include protection against free radicals, cardiovascular and nervous system diseases, strengthening of bones and joints, and improvement of brain, liver, pancreas, and digestive functions. However, since RTD teas frequently contain lower levels of dried tea leaves and buds, called "tea solids," and fewer polyphenols because their base ingredient may not be brewed tea, the benefits are generally fewer and less concentrated than they are in brewed tea. This is according to a study performed by C. Cabreera, R. Giménez, and C. López in the *Journal of Agricultural and Food Chemistry*. Also some people object to the sugar because of the added calories and potential for causing tooth decay.

Tea Liqueurs

One chic way to take tea these days is in a cocktail. Yet as everything old has a way of coming around to being new again, mixing alcohol and tea has long been enjoyed by many cultures worldwide, especially in England. Since the nineteenth century and even before, people have been concocting hot toddies to warm their bones on cold, blustery nights. A hot toddy combines hot tea with whiskey or rum, honey, and spices.

Nowadays consumers prefer tea liqueurs made from neutral spirits infused with powdered green tea, herbs, and sugar. Companies that produce spirits are cashing in on the desire of the hip, younger consumer to indulge in alcohol but at the same time slim down, lower cholesterol, quaff some antioxidants, and perhaps also bring a little peace, harmony, and cheer to after-work relaxation. Tea purists mostly agree that the subtle aroma and taste of tea in such drinks is obliterated by the strong alcohol flavor. The health benefits of the tea in tea liqueurs is counterbalanced by the high amounts of sugar and alcohol used in preparation.

Iced Tea

In spite of the above mentioned trends, by far the most common way Americans take their tea is iced. Around 85 percent of the tea we consume is iced tea, and Americans drink it year round. The majority of ice tea you find in conventional restaurants will be black, but specialty coffee shops and others are expanding to include green and herbal iced teas.

Exactly who and when iced tea was invented remains suspended in the glaciers of time, but the custom seems to have come into fashion sometime during the nineteenth century in both the US and in Britain as an extension of popular alcoholic green tea punches. The trend, however, did not continue in Britain as it has in the US. The rise in consumption of nonalcoholic iced tea parallels the invention of refrigeration (1876) and the introduction of refrigerators into the average home. Although consumers were already drinking iced tea, it hit big at the 1904 St. Louis World's Fair. During that scorching summer, Richard Blechynden, director of the East Indian Pavilion, offered tea with ice to quench attendees' thirsty palates. Prohibition in the 1920s gave both tea and coffee a boost because these drinks provided refreshing nonalcoholic alternatives. Iced tea paraphernalia such as tall tea glasses, long spoons, and lemon forks were widespread by 1930. Then during World War II, when America's green tea supply from Japan was cut off (at the time, Japan produced almost all of the green tea sold on the world market), Americans turned to drinking black iced tea, which was produced in India and distributed under British supervision.

Sweet Tea

Sweet tea has been a favorite thirst quencher throughout the South since the nineteenth century, and the trend is still going strong today. In spite of the cold weather, many Canadians also drink sweet tea with their meals, and the beverage is readily available from supermarkets in the US. Sweet tea, since it is made of tea, carries the same health benefits of other teas. The addition of sugar infuses the body with an added spurt of energy and plenty of carbohydrates.

Tea and Color Healing

The color of any food or drink exerts profound psychological and physical effects on the human body, and tea is no exception. The idea that different food colors affect people psychologically did not originate with nouvelle cuisine. Color has been recognized for its therapeutic values throughout history. Cultures as different as Native American, Middle Eastern, Celtic, Central Asian, Chinese, Druidic, Greek, and Teutonic all used it. Ancient Egyptians even constructed color halls at Karnack and Thebes where they researched color therapy and performed healings using color.

In modern times, an entire field dedicated to the study of color psychology and color therapy has emerged. Chromotherapists, that is, healers who use color to cure ailments, believe that disease indicates an imbalance at one or more levels of the physical and spiritual bodies. These bodies reputedly are linked to energy centers in the body known as chakras.

Under normal circumstances, each chakra absorbs light and filters the colors needed to feed the organism.

An energy blockage occurs when one or more chakras are prohibited from filtering and processing the ideal color frequencies. The result is disharmony in the system, which can lead to illness and disease. To restore balance, chromotherapists sometimes beam colored light on the afflicted areas. They may also prescribe a diet of foods of specific colors and/or certain teas and herbal teas. To clarify this concept, the following three paragraphs show how chromotherapy works with fruit and vegetables.

Fruit and vegetables contain natural pigments that are both visually appealing and provide nutrition. The concept that everyone should eat a rainbow of colors daily from produce in order to achieve and maintain good health is a growing trend. For example, according to chromotherapists, a red sauce made from tomatoes protects against heart disease and cancers, especially of the prostate. The orange beta carotene in acorn squash soup strengthens the immune system and helps keep the eyes in youthful shape. The blueberries in a smoothie contain the powerful antioxidant anthocyanin, which can improve memory and reduce the risk of heart disease and stroke.

Where the psychology of color enters the scene has to do with the patient's attitude toward what is being consumed. If one believes that the color of the food or drink will help cure a malady, the natural effect will probably be enhanced. This is not exactly a placebo effect, because the substances do contain ingredients with proven therapeutic effects, but the patient is helping the result along by keeping an open, positive attitude.

When looking at the colors of tea, more variables come into play. A tea's tint depends somewhat on climate, altitude, soil where the tea is grown, weather conditions, and where and how it is processed by different producers at different times. Lightly oxidized tea is greener and the more heavily oxidized variety is redder. Even within these variations, tea can exert constant, measurable effects on the body. Every tea or herbal tea will have some color to it. Even single-ingredient teas and herbal teas come in diverse colors. There are five basic tea colors: white (which often melds into yellow), green, orange, red, and brown. There is black, too, but that usually happens when tea is brewed too strongly.

In general, white teas are relaxing, and can be imbibed for spiritual goals, for example, to enhance a meditation experience. Green represents balance of body, mind, and spirit. Green teas are often drunk to improve health. Not every green tea looks green in the cup. It may be yellow-colored as is yellow tea. Black teas, which when brewed often turn mahogany red or orangey amber, increase energy and alertness. Not coincidentally, they also contain the most caffeine. According to chromotherapists, brown-hued teas can help eliminate indecisiveness, improve concentration, and awaken the digestive system. Examples of such teas are many black varieties, kuan yin, which looks brownish-green in the cup, and puerhs. In the herbal tea department, roasted dandelion root makes a clear brown color in the teacup.

No matter the color, all teas and herbal teas should look clear and bright in the cup. More information on the colors of specific tea and their uses in healing is provided in succeeding chapters.

Two

Black Tea

This chapter discusses black tea and lists some popular varieties with descriptions of what they do healthwise. Black tea has many health benefits. It can stimulate the nerve cells of the brain to make a certain protein that delays the onset of dementia and Alzheimer's, improve memory, and increase alertness. Black tea also contains flavonoids. Flavonoids are an antioxidant that can reduce the likelihood that a person can contract esophageal cancer. One useful study on the flavonoids in black tea was written by C. Cabrera, R. Giménez, and M. C. López, published in the *Journal of Agricultural and Food Chemistry.*

Here are some other health benefits that have been studied having to do with consumption of black tea. In this chapter, one source of information is listed after each benefit. Complete data on the sources is listed in the Reference section of this book.

- **Fosters alertness**—Because black tea contains caffeine and another stimulating substance called theophylline, it can speed up heart rate to make the drinker feel more alert. (E.A. de Bruin, J. J. Rowson, L. Van Buren, J. A. Rycroft, *Appetite*).

- **Lowers risk of diabetes**—(A. Beresniak, G. Duru, G. Berger, D. Bremond-Gignac, *BMJ Open)*.

- **Prevents arteries from clogging**—(J. A. Vinson, K. Teufel, N. Wu, *Journal of Agriculture and Food Chemistry)*.

- **Lowers risk of kidney stones**—(G. C. Curhan, W. C. Willett, F. E. Speozer. K. K. Stamfer. *Annals of Internal Medicine)*.

- **Boosts metabolism to facilitate weight loss**—(B. G. Pollock, M. Wylie, J. A. Stack et al., *Journal of Clinical Pharmacology)*.

- **Raise blood pressure**—For those who suffer from low blood pressure.

- **Protects against prostate cancer**—(L. Jian, A. H. Lee, C. W. Bins, *Asian Pacific Journal of Clinical Nutrition)*.

- **Protects against osteoporosis**—(O. Johnell, B. L. Gullberg, J. A. Kanis, *Journal of Bone Mineral Research*).

- **Helps attenuate symptoms of Parkinson's Disease**—(H. Checkoway, K. Powers, T. Smith-Weller, et al., *American Journal of Epidemiology*).

- **Protects against lung cancer**—(N. Tang, Y. Wu. B; Zhou, B. Wang, R. Yu, *Lung Cancer)*.

- **Helps lower LDL cholesterol**—(J. M. Davoes. J. T. Judd, D. J. Bieretal, *Journal of Nutrition*).

- **Protects against ovarian cancer**—(B. Zhou, Yang L., Wang L., et al., *American Journal of Obstetrics and Gynecology)*.

Not included in the list but deserving mention is the calming effect of tea on body and mind due to the presence of theophylline as well as the phytonutrients tea adds to the diet.

Black Tea and Color Healing

Because some black teas can look mahogany red in the cup, they are sometimes associated with this hue in color healing. The color red represents energy, enthusiasm, good health, strength, willpower, courage, intensity, war, love, passion, and virility. Shades of all colors create subtle changes in the kind of energy they bring to tea. Drink red-colored teas to strengthen your constitution after an illness and to free yourself from the lingering psychological effects of a recent illness. A few herbal teas are also red in color; rooibos, honeybush, hibiscus, and rosehips are examples.

Other black teas look somewhat orange in the cup. Orange-colored teas help clear and revitalize the intellect. They also enjoy a reputation as vision-enhancers. They can recharge left brain batteries, enhance self-control, and stimulate willpower and the ability to adapt to circumstances. They also help a person declutter and organize the closet of the mind. These brews may even motivate one to achieve success. The superb-tasting orange pekoe, even though it was named for the Royal House of Holland and not because of its color, is a prime example. In the herbal tea category, calendula fits the bill.

Caffeine, Tannins, and Black Tea

There can also be some negative and even harmful effects to drinking tea, especially black tea. Consumption of black tea can aggravate fibrocystic disease if you already suffer from it, and those prone to acne, especially teenagers, can experience breakouts after consuming black tea. Tea can cause diarrhea and tremors in caffeine-sensitive people. If your serum potassium levels are abnormally low, you should not drink any kind of tea at all.

Besides these potential medical issues, you need to consider tea's caffeine content, which is greatest in black tea than in other types of tea. The caffeine in black tea can accelerate heartbeat and raise blood pressure. This is good for maintaining alertness and for helping people with low blood pressure, but it can also be harmful if you have high blood pressure or coronary issues. Other side effects of drinking black tea are anxiety, headache, increased urination, insomnia, irregular heartbeat, nausea and vomiting, nervousness, restlessness, ringing in the ears, and tremors. These side effects have been reported in the journal *Molecular Aspects of Medicine*, among other places.

It is true that a pound of dried black tea contains twice the caffeine of a pound of coffee. However, you can brew approximately two hundred cups of fairly strong tea from that pound compared to around forty cups of coffee, making the caffeine content of the coffee you drink much denser than what is found in tea. From the USDA National Nutrient Database for Standard Reference comes the following list of caffeine amounts for different types of brewed teas:

- **White tea, 8 ounces**—15 mg

- **Green tea, 8 ounces**—20 mg

- **Oolong tea, 8 ounces**—30 mg

- **Black tea, 8 ounces**—48 mg

- **Black coffee, 8 ounces**—135–140 mg

Luckily, tea also contains the mild muscle relaxants theophylline and theobromine, which naturally help neutralize the negative aspects of caffeine. By indulging in a cup or two, you can remain alert and relaxed. Of course your overall health and individual tolerance for caffeine plays a large role in determining how much tea you can drink. If you cannot tolerate any caffeine at all, then herbal teas may be the route for you to go instead. Except for yerba mate, which contains more caffeine than black tea, they are caffeine-free.

You may also want to drink decaffeinated tea. As with coffee, there are several methods of decaffeination. Unfortunately, some manufacturers remove the caffeine with ethyl acetate, a highly flammable solvent that's in nail polish. Even in residual amounts, this chemical is a skin irritant that can also cause sore throats, cough, dizziness, headache, and nausea. Environmentally aware manufacturers like Celestial Seasonings have chosen to decaffeinate using carbon dioxide and water, which is a perfectly safe process. The more naturally tea is decaffeinated, the more antioxidants and flavor are retained. Be advised that many decaffeinated teas taste dull. Decaf tea, it seems, does not interact as favorably with the tannins, essential oils, and polyphenols, which create the rich and varied palette of tea fragrances and flavors.

Decaffeination

You can eliminate half of the caffeine in your cup of tea by performing what is known as a "second potting." Since caffeine dissolves in boiling water, decaffeinate your tea by removing the leaves from the pot after steeping and transferring them to a second, empty pot. Pour boiling water over the leaves again, steep once more, and you will have reduced the amount of caffeine contained in the tea by approximately 50 percent.

Tannins and Black Tea

Contrary to popular belief, the tannins in tea are not the tannic acid used to cure leather. They are a subgroup of antioxidants consisting of natural chemical compounds called catechins. Catechins are a type of polyphenol found in many vegetables and fruit. Both red wine and tea contain tannins, which interact with the proteins of the mouth to lend the uniquely astringent taste to these beverages. Black tea contains the highest percentage of tannins, but green tea, especially a hearty green tea like gunpowder, and some herbal teas like yerba mate also have them. Just one infused cup of green tea contains 200 mg of catechins, while you would need to drink a liter of wine to come up with 300 mg.

The same astringency that gives tea its flavor also functions as an antiseptic and antioxidant to help the stomach digest fatty foods. Tannins also help ward off bacteria and alkaloid poisoning from substances that contain, for example, ephedra, ergot (a grain fungus), nicotine, or strychnine. Research has shown that tea's tannins can strengthen the immune system and cause cancer cells to self-destruct. In addition, they can lessen the damage done to lipids and DNA during digestion and keep the body from absorbing cholesterol. A few studies have shown that tea may have the potential to prevent coronary artery disease, heart attack and stroke as well. Research into these areas continues, but more needs to be done before any of the above claims can be stated as absolute facts.

What is known about the tannins in tea is that they can interfere with the body's absorption of iron. This is according to the Natural Medicines Comprehensive Database on black tea. Those who are anemic, vegan, or vegetarian should limit their tea consumption to three cups per day and not drink it with meals. Black tea's tannins can also inhibit absorption of certain medications such as tricyclics antidepressants. If you are especially sensitive to tannins, you may find that tea irritates your bowels, kidneys, and even your liver.

If you wish to cut down on the tannins in your tea and you are not lactose intolerant, try adding some milk. Instead of binding to the proteins in your mouth, the tannins will attack the milk's proteins. You will lessen the tannins but miss out on the antioxidants and great tea taste.

Types of Black Tea

Numerous possible single black teas and blends are available on the market today. The following lists a few bestsellers with short descriptions and some suggested health benefits:

- **Assam**—More black tea comes from this state in India than from anywhere else. Assam teas have a pleasant malty aroma. If alertness is what you desire, Assam will keep you awake because it contains a lot of caffeine.

- **Ceylon**—Grown in Sri Lanka (formerly known as Ceylon), this bright orange-colored tea in the cup exudes a flowery aroma and light aftertaste. Ceylon supplies the base for many blends. Ceylon tea, as well as all other teas, can tone your cardiovascular system.

- **Constant Comment**—A spicy recipe originally from Colonial America and refined by Ruth Campbell Bigelow in the 1940s, it is a black tea flavored with orange peel, cinnamon, and clove. This zesty tea is still produced by the Bigelow Tea Company and ranks as the number-one selling flavored black tea in the US. As with other teas, it can help improve memory and invigorate the body.

- **Darjeeling**—A full-bodied, amber-colored liquid with a pleasing flowery, fresh taste. It is cultivated at altitudes of around seven thousand feet in the Himalayas. Darjeeling is called the "champagne of teas" both for its exceptional taste and because it is so difficult to harvest. Drink Darjeeling as well as other teas to improve digestion.

- **Earl Grey**—As the story goes, this blend is a once secret formula given to a British Prime Minister by an Imperial Chinese mandarin in gratitude for a successful diplomatic mission. Earl grey blends china black and Darjeeling teas and is scented with citrusy oil of bergamot. The citrus adds a bit of vitamin C to this tea to strengthen the immune system.

- **English Breakfast**—A brisk, full-bodied, colorful blend of Chinese keemun and Yunnan province blacks, Indian, and ceylon teas. As is the case with other black teas, English breakfast tea is drunk to stimulate the brain, especially in the morning.

- **Irish Breakfast**—This is a strong black tea drunk to maintain mental alertness.

- **Keemun**—Formerly known as China Imperial tea, this fine-grade, hand-rolled, and fired black tea from China's Anhui province exudes a spicy, slightly toasty bouquet. Quality varies according to the year's harvest. As with the other types of tea, keemun is drunk to ease the digestion.

- **Lapsang Souchong**—A Chinese tea black fired over pine root logs to give it a smoky aroma and taste. It can be drunk to improve memory.

- **Orange Pekoe**—Many people mistakenly think that orange pekoe (pronounced "peck-oh") is a type of scented tea. The term actually refers to a large-leaf tea that, when first introduced to the West, was marketed as the preferred tea of the Dutch Royal House of Orange. When fully oxidized and brewed, it displays a bright orange color. It is drunk, as are most teas, to improve digestion.

Three

Green Tea

This chapter discusses the health benefits of green tea and lists the most popular varieties with a description of what they do, health wise. It also includes a short section on scented teas.

As you learned in chapter 1, green tea leaves are only lightly oxidized. Green tea contains very few tannins and little caffeine—less than 10 percent of the caffeine content of coffee. While this is good for healthy living, the flavor is impacted. You will not find a green tea whose flavor approaches the robust spiciness of fully oxidized black teas that you may be accustomed to. On the other hand, this makes it easy to add floral and fruit scents to enhance green teas' subtle aromas and flavors, leading to an almost infinite variety of intriguing combinations. Scented teas are discussed at the end of this chapter.

As with wines, tea tasters employ many exotic terms to describe green tea flavors. For example, they characterize a tea as tasting like asparagus, bamboo, bittersweet, butter, cocoa, cut grass, flower, fruit, green bean, melon, mushroom, nut, field pea, pine, seaweed, spinach, swamp (!), vegetal, or vanilla bean. Later in this chapter, some of the more popular varietals and how you can expect them to taste are listed. Since this book is for beginners, the various tastes will be described in simpler terms.

At first, green tea was consumed in Asia with the conviction that it improved health and well-being. Tea was not drunk socially among all classes in China until around the fifteenth century. As was stated in chapter 1, green tea was the first type imported to the West in 1610 by the Dutch from Japan as a health drink. It was also fairly well-liked in the US until World War II. During the war, the supply of Japanese green tea, which was the only exporter of green tea at the time, was cut off, and so the US began getting tea from India via the British. After the war, it seems that green tea all but disappeared from Americans' collective radar to be replaced by the ever-popular coffee.

Today, green tea is back in favor. Over the past decade with the rise of China's and other Asian or Eastern economies, interest has been rekindled in all things from these countries, including food and drink. Eastern-style meditation, religions, martial arts, yoga, and Asian or Eastern health cures, including the use of certain herbs and teas have filtered into American culture, supported by promotions from celebrities and health gurus.

Many Americans are on the lookout for a miracle cure—one that's easy on the wallet and a pleasure to consume, and green tea seems to fit the bill. It has been touted as a healthy drink that cures everything from high cholesterol to cancer. Reams of research papers have been written about the health benefits of green tea, and time after time, they show promising results. Noted researcher in the field of tea, Dr. Thomas G. Sherman, Associate Professor in the Department of Pharmacology and Physiology at Georgetown University Medical Center, says that he is astounded by the fact that the more tea you drink, the better it is for you (the complete reference is listed at the end of this book). So why is the ability of green tea to affect the human organism in a positive way still an issue? As with most complex topics, the answer is not simple.

In the first place, a significant number of the investigations have been performed in the laboratory exclusively with animals, mainly mice. While human studies have been done, as often as not, the researchers have not separated the effects of tea consumption from general diet and lifestyle. Some have not monitored the amount and concentration of green tea that the subjects consumed. A few have not even indicated whether the green tea consumption was taken as a beverage, pill, extract, food, or by some other method. Sometimes only a general correlation between green tea consumption and health benefits is verified and researchers still are not certain of the amounts that can be absorbed by the body. Some researchers (including the above quoted Dr. Sherman) love tea, but are not certain whether to attribute the results of the experiments to the antioxidants present in the tea, to other components or to combinations of components. Therefore, organizations like the National Institute of Health conclude that there is not enough evidence to determine green tea's benefits.

Green tea contains EGCG. EGCG is an acronym for epigallocatechin-3-gallate, a catechin, a class of polyphenols. Polyphenols are molecules that possess potent antioxidant properties. EGCG is present in some fruit and vegetables and abounds in green tea. In fact, one eight-ounce cup of green tea contains as many antioxidants as one cup of blueberries. EGCG is particularly concentrated in green tea because it is processed without being fermented; that is, oxidation is minimal. (Source: C. Cabrera, R. Giménez, M. C. López, *Journal of Agricultural and Food Chemistry.*)

Although the National Cancer Institute does not recommend for or against consumption of green tea to reduce the risk of any type of cancer, the ability of the EGCG in green tea to interfere with the growth of cancers of the bladder, colon, esophagus, liver, lung, ovaries, pancreas, prostate and stomach has been studied with some promising results. One such study was performed by H. Mukhtar and N. Ahmed concerning tea's polyphenols and their role in cancer prevention and health optimization. This study was reported in the *American Journal of Clinical Nutrition*. A study by Q. Li, M. Kakizaki, S. Kuriyama, et al. and published in the *British Journal of Cancer*, is also quite positive as to the effect of green tea on the liver.

Unfortunately, the results of studies exploring the ability of green tea to prevent breast cancer have been inconclusive. Several studies have borne out this conclusion, including a case-control study in Southeast China performed by M. Zhang, C. D. Holman, J. P. Huang, and X. Xie, published in the journal *Carcinogenesis*.

Researchers at Harvard and other institutions have shown that green tea reduces the risk of hearth attack and stroke by lowering levels of LDL (bad) cholesterol that clog arteries. One such study that backs this claim was published in the *Journal of Agricultural and Food Chemistry* by researchers from the University of Scranton, Scranton, PA, J. A. Vinson, K. Teufel, and N. Wu. The combination of catechins and fluoride in green tea has been found to strengthen the teeth by killing off bacteria that cause tooth decay and gum disease. In an interview with WebMD, Christine D. Wu, Ph.D., a microbiologist and professor of periodontics at the University of Illinois at the Chicago College of Dentistry, confirms that according to her extensive research in the field, the polyphenols in green tea "prevent bacterial growth…and fight infection and even cavities." The catechins along with the anti-inflammatory properties and phytoestrogens present in green tea also help fortify bones by retarding skeletal breakdown while at the same time building more bone cells. One such study that bolsters this claim was performed by C. Shen, J. K. Yeh, J. J. Cao, and J. S. Wang from the Department of Pathology at Texas Tech and published in the *Nutrition Research* journal.

It seems that green tea may also lubricate the gray matter of the brain. Clinical trials are currently being undertaken at Taipei Hospital in Taiwan to study the capacity of green tea to inhibit type-2 diabetes by regulating glucose levels. Studies as to green tea's ability to slow the progress of neurological disorders like Alzheimer's, Parkinson's, and Crohn's by strengthening cognitive abilities also look hopeful. One such study comes from the Tohoku University Graduate School of Medicine in Sendai, Japan was performed by S. Kuriyama, A. Hozawa, K. Ohmori, et al. and published in the *American Journal of Clinical Nutrition*. Researchers in this area are focusing on a specific amino acid found in green tea leaves called L-Theanine. This amino acid is said to affect the central nervous system by producing a sense of calmness and clarity.

Consumption of green tea is also associated with lessening the chance for men to contract prostate cancer. This is according to a study, among others, performed by N. Kurahashi, S. Sasazuki, M. Iwasaki, and S. Tsugane concerning prostate cancer risk in Japanese men and green tea consumption, which was published in the *American Journal of Epidemiology*.

The jury is still out on the ability of consumption of green tea to promote weight loss, but some studies show potential. One such study by T. Nagao, T. Hase, and I. Tokimitsu was published in the journal *Obesity*. Such studies point to the ability of the catechins found in green tea to produce enough body heat, known to scientists as "thermogenesis," to raise metabolism, oxidize fat, and burn more calories. Three cups of green tea per day is the recommended dose.

To shed a few extra pounds it is recommended that a person eat less and exercise more. In addition, you can start the day by quaffing a big mug of green tea. Before drinking, liberally squeeze the juice from a fresh lemon slice into your brew. The tea and lemon act together to help flush toxins that have built up in your body overnight. To help suppress your appetite throughout the day, drink a steaming cup of green tea and lemon before each meal. Spice up this tea with cardamom and fennel seeds and stir with a cinnamon stick. The spices will kill off your appetite and sweeten the tea in the bargain. Finally, before retiring, instead of snacking, sip a bedtime cup of your favorite green tea without the lemon or spices.

Green Tea and Color Healing

Some green teas look green when they are brewed in the cup, and therefore are associated with this hue in color healing. The predominant color of nature, green also stands in a harmonious position between the red and blue ends of the color spectrum. In symbolic terms, it is the quintessential hue of prosperity, good luck, abundance, success, and rejuvenation. As a color that represents equanimity, peace, and harmony, green-colored teas can be drunk to help heal the spirit and make a happy home. As to the body, color healers maintain that green-colored teas help put out-of-whack systems back into balance.

Mother Nature has provided humans with a bounty of healthy, emerald-colored teas. Among them are gyokuro, sencha, and matcha, as well as peppermint and spearmint herbal teas.

Other green teas exhibit a clear yellow color when brewed. Since most white teas (white tea is a kind of green tea) appear yellow in the cup, this hue is discussed along with white teas in chapter 4.

There is a flipside to drinking green tea. In spite of the health advantages associated with it, green tea can interfere with certain medications. If you take blood thinners, the recommendation is to consult your physician or pharmacist before drinking this kind of tea. If your serum potassium levels are abnormally low, you should not drink tea. If you are not sure about the interaction between green tea and the medication you are taking, consult your physician or pharmacist before drinking green tea.

Although green tea contains many fewer tannins than its black counterpart, it is not tannin-free. Vegetarians, vegans, or those suffering from anemia may need to limit their green tea intake or, at the very least, not drink it with meals because it may hamper absorption of iron and vitamin B. Because green tea contains some caffeine and tannins, pregnant and nursing women are advised to avoid it, especially during early stages of pregnancy. Finally, the fluoride found in green tea that can combat tooth decay in very few cases can also cause a condition known as "fluorosis." This condition can cause mottling of the teeth as well as bone fractures, especially in children and patients with bone diseases. For a healthy adult, however, it would take steady consumption of green tea over such a long a period to acquire this condition.

Green Tea Extracts

Another way to ingest green tea besides drinking it as a beverage is to consume green tea extracts. An extract is a plant preparation of a liquid or viscous consistency usually soaked in alcohol that delivers a strong, concentrated dose of the substance. An extract may contain one or more botanical substances. Extracts can be used in both cooking and herbal medicine. Sometimes an extract is made from a tea or herb(s) with the intention of delivering more potent therapeutic benefits than can be obtained by drinking the beverage or by swallowing a capsule. Because green tea extracts draw out the distilled essence of the leaf and bud, they taste bitter. Green tea extract is drunk principally to lose weight, fight infection, brighten overall health, improve glucose tolerance, and alleviate insulin resistance in those suffering from type-2 diabetes.

Be aware that since an extract delivers a stronger dose of catechins, caffeine, and tannins than beverage green tea, it can cause insomnia, nausea, digestive, and thyroid problems, and in extreme cases abdominal spasms and heart palpitations. These troubles usually surface with longterm overconsumption. However, even moderate consumption of green tea extracts can cause an allergic reaction such as itchy skin and rash.

If you want to buy green tea extracts, the suggestion is to shop around for a good, reliable brand, preferably one offered at a natural health food store or natural grocery rather than through the Internet. Salespeople at brick-and-mortar stores tend to be knowledgeable and picky about the brands they carry to satisfy their customers. No matter where you purchase your green tea extract, make sure it is made from real tea and that it contains no additives such as fillers.

To be absolutely certain you are consuming a pure extract, you may prefer to prepare your own. To do this you will usually use the leaf, flower, and/or bud of the plant. Put four ounces of dried or eight ounces of fresh, bruised herbs into a 16-ounce dark-colored bottle. The bottle's dark color helps slow deterioration from light. The most commonly found colors are brown, cobalt blue, or green.

Fill the rest of the bottle with grain alcohol, vodka, or gin. Substitute vinegar if you prefer a nonalcoholic preparation, but keep in mind the taste will be like vinegar. Add three or four drops of food grade vitamin E as a preservative.

Cap the bottle and shake well. Store the extract in a cool, dry place away from the sun. A basement or root cellar shelf is ideal.

Shake the bottle twice a day for three to twenty-one days until you have achieved the desired strength. Then uncap the bottle and pour the mixture into another bottle through cheesecloth or a coffee filter to remove the botanicals. Your result will be something between a tincture and a true extract in strength, ready to consume. Ten to thirty drops per day is an average recommended dose, depending on the extract's strength. Keep refrigerated.

Brassica Tea

Before moving on to the list of different kinds of green tea, one type is worthy of special mention. Brassica tea is described here separately because its components are especially good for healthy living. Brassica tea has many health benefits because it also contains a component found in broccoli. That said, very little of the broccoli flavor, if any, makes it into brassica tea.

More than a decade ago, scientists from Johns Hopkins University isolated the antioxidant in broccoli that battles free radicals and keeps them from destroying cells in the body, which can open the door to cancer and other chronic conditions. They called their find "sulforaphane" or SGS for short. Researchers were able to extract SGS from broccoli and add it to tea. Although any kind of tea can be infused with SGS, it seems to harmonize best with the vegetal flavors of various green teas.

Just one cup of brassica tea will deliver to your body the equivalent of three ounces of fresh broccoli. You bypass the distinctive broccoli taste and get an added nutritional boost courtesy of green tea's catechins. This is why some enthusiasts believe brassica tea may be the healthiest tea on the planet.

Brassica tea can be purchased online at baltcoffee .com, amazon.com, greenmarket.com, and internatural .com. It can also be bought at most Whole Foods stores, some Trader Joe's, at Baltimore Coffee and Tea stores, and at Wegman stores in the American northeast. For complete information on the history and health benefits of brassica tea, visit their website at www.brassica.com.

Common Types of Green Tea

This chapter moves on to common types of green tea and what they do health wise. One must understand that all green teas do more or less the same thing health wise because they are all the same tea. Some variation in vitamin and mineral content, caffeine and tannin amounts as well as pollutants do occur. These differences are due to growing conditions and regions where the tea is cultivated, and slight variations in processing techniques. Hundreds of varieties of green teas are available on the market today. The following list describes kinds you are likely to find on your natural grocery and health food store shelves. First, the name of the tea is stated, then its alternative name and country of origin to help you when you ask for it in a store or online. This is followed by a short description of each tea and a suggested health benefit.

- **Bancha (Japan)**—Unlike most green teas, the coarse leaves are picked late in the season and harvested together with the stems and stalks to make bancha. Tea masters will tell you that this brew tastes flat, but the Japanese drink it as a daily tea in the same way Americans might drink Lipton's black. To give bancha its due, it is cheaper than the higher grade teas and pairs well with most foods. Another advantage is that it delivers a generous dose of digestive enzymes. Therefore, a major health benefit of bancha is to aid digestion.

- **Dragonwell (also Lung Ching; China)**—The flat and shiny leaf of this acclaimed tea with its sweet, smooth flavor is among the earliest known Chinese teas. There are six quality grades of Dragonwell; the best is hand-tossed in special iron pans. The liquid appears clear yellow, almost citrine-like. Therefore, it can represent the yellow hue in color healing. Dragonwell rose to fame during the time in American history when it was presented to President Nixon on his celebrated visit to China. As with all green teas, Dragonwell is thought to help mitigate cancers such as of the esophagus.

- **Genmaicha (also spelled Gen Mai Cha; Japan)**—This nutty, crispy tasting green sencha tea is sometimes called "popcorn tea" because the toasted rice with which it is mixed sometimes makes popping noises in the cup. It is considered a good choice to serve to those whose palates are not familiar with green tea. The leaves are pan-fired before being combined with the toasted rice. Since genmaicha is a sencha tea, the health benefits are the same as for sencha tea (see below).

- **Gunpowder (also Pearl Tea; China)**—This green tea grown primarily in Zhanjiang province has been drunk in China since the Tang Dynasty (618–907). The name comes from the way the blend of new and old grayish-green leaves is rolled to resemble gunpowder pellets or little pearls in shape and color. Small, tightly rolled pellets mark a better quality tea than the larger pellets. Gunpowder's flavor is robust, almost like a black tea. This is due to the way it is processed with more oxidation than most greens. Consequently, it also contains more caffeine. Because gunpowder tea contains more caffeine, it is a good tea to drink to stay alert. Gunpowder tea is also thought to promote weight loss, as are other green, black, yellow, and white teas.

- **Gyokuro (Japan)**—The bushes of this superior quality tea are shaded by awnings during the last twenty days before harvesting. Keeping the leaves away from direct sunlight makes them produce more chlorophyll, resulting in a sweetly fragranced bouquet with a pure, vegetal taste. The flat, sharply pointed leaves look green in the brewed cup. Because the leaves are shaded, they retain a high concentration of amino acids and other nutrients. Because amino acids are the building blocks for forming protein, people who are deficient in protein, such as some vegetarians and vegans, can benefit from drinking Gyokuro tea.

- **Houjicha (also spelled Hojicha; Japan)**—This tea receives its reddish-brown color, deep aroma, and nutty taste from roasting the large, flat leaves over charcoal. The procedure results in less caffeine than most green teas. Houjicha makes a good choice for tea drinkers who are sensitive to caffeine. Like all green teas, houjicha makes a reasonable tea to drink to help prevent bladder cancer.

- **Matcha (also spelled Maccha; Japan)**—The Japanese powder this shade-grown tea from the Fuji region and use it in their tea ceremony, a cultural tradition that lies outside the purview of this book. For a description of the Japanese tea ceremony, it is recommended that you visit sites such as www.teavana.com/tea-info/japanese-tea -ceremony. Following tradition, producers crush the leaves in a stone mill. Since the entire leaf is powdered, the amino acids and nutrients are especially potent in this tea. While it contains more caffeine than most greens, matcha also has a fair amount of the amino acid L-theanine, a natural relaxant. Therefore, it is a good tea to drink in order to relax. Because of the concentration of amino acids in this tea, people who suffer from bone, tooth, or hair loss can drink it to positive effect.

- **Pi Lo Chun tea (also spelled Bi Luo Chun; China)**— This popular green tea's name means "Green Snail Spring." The name refers to the way this tea is rolled into a tight spiral that resembles a snail shell. Mainly it is grown in the slightly acidic soil of Zhejiang province of China amidst apricot, peach, and plum trees. As the fruit trees burst into bloom, the tender new tea shoots absorb the sweet aroma wafting through the air. You can sample this tea anytime, but during the spring is especially appropriate because pi lo chun enhances the flavors and health benefits of springtime dishes. As with all green teas, pi lo chun may be drunk to boost the immune system.

- **Pouchong (Taiwan)**—This tea from the Wenshan region is so named for the way the Cantonese used to package it in little paper packets. The flavor is mild enough that the tea is often found blended with scented teas and stronger green teas. Rose pouchong is an especially delectable scented tea. The rose blossoms with which this tea is scented will add a trace of vitamin C, so it can be drunk to bolster the immune system.

- **Sencha (Japan)**—Like bancha, sencha is drunk daily by the Japanese. But sencha is generally a first-rate tea that is better than bancha. The best quality sencha tastes fresh and tangy and the color is a bright emerald green, and so is allied with the green hue in color healing. Because sencha leaves are exposed to a good deal of sunlight, the leaves manufacture a significant amount of catechins. Those who subscribe to color healing drink sencha tea to detoxify the body.

- **Twig Tea (also Kuki Cha; Japan)**—Twig tea is produced from the white stems, one bud and three leaves of the tea plant. This tea exudes an earthy aroma and woody, chestnut-like flavor. It contains almost no caffeine; therefore it is a good tea for caffeine-sensitive people to drink. Like all green teas, twig tea helps manage cholesterol levels.

- **White Monkey Paw (China)**—Despite its name, this is a green tea. The top two leaves and bud of the new season's growth are plucked so early they still retain their downy "hair." The taste is exceptionally light. Men might want to drink this type of tea to lessen their risk of contracting prostate cancer.

- **Young Hyson (China)**—"Hyson" (or xichun) in Mandarin means "flourishing spring." Young Hyson refers to the very first leaves that are harvested before the rainy season sets in. This premium China tea's greenish-yellow leaves are thinly rolled so that they appear twisted. Young Hyson has a bolder, more full-bodied flavor than most green teas, yet it still tastes warm and smooth. This type of tea is thought to be especially helpful for weight loss for both men and women. Be sure to look for the young varietal, as regular hyson is of middling quality.

No matter what kind of green tea you choose, you will need to steep it differently from black, oolong, and herbal teas. To learn the best ways to brew green tea as well as others, see chapter 7, which is dedicated to how to brew tea.

Not everybody enjoys the taste of green tea—at least, not initially. One way to accustom oneself to the grassy taste is to start with gunpowder green, described earlier. Because this tea is more oxidized than other greens, its taste more readily approximates the black teas you may be accustomed to drinking.

Scented Green Teas

Another way to get acquainted with the nuanced flavors of green tea is through scented teas. Asians have been scenting their teas for centuries. If you have ever eaten at a Chinese or Vietnamese restaurant, undoubtedly you have drunk green tea scented with jasmine blossoms, a staple served in such establishments.

Due to its subtle flavor, green tea takes scenting especially well, although blacks, such as Earl Grey, and oolongs also can be successfully scented. To scent a tea, fresh flower petals as well as fruits, spices, and even fruit peels are added to the leaves during the final drying stage. When the scented elements are removed, their delicate aroma and taste lingers. A scented tea, besides tasting good, has a slight advantage over plain green tea in that it infuses the liquid with extra, albeit miniscule, amounts of vitamins and other nutrients.

Along with jasmine, popular scents for teas include bergamot, chamomile, cherry blossom, cinnamon, clove bud, chrysanthemum flowers, fennel, gardenia, ginger, hibiscus, kiwi, lavender, lemon, lime, lychee, marigold, mint, narcissus, orange, peach tree leaf, rose, saffron, vanilla bean, and violet.

Sometimes the scent is added in the form of essential oils. If you buy tea scented with oils, verify that the oil is a true essence. That is to say, make sure it is the pure oil extracted from the plant, not a synthetic concocted in a laboratory, which can be harmful to your health.

Sometimes more than one flavor is infused into the green tea. Such teas are delicious served over ice on hot summer days. One example of how flavor and health benefits merge is lemon ginger green tea. The mild green tea flavor blends well with the spicy warmth of ginger and the citrus of lemon and lemongrass. The ginger is beneficial for dieting, flatulent colic, diarrhea, kidney trouble, and chest complaints. Another good example is snow blossom tea. This tea mingles green tea with chamomile, rose, jasmine, and lavender blossoms for an exquisite summer bouquet. The chamomile helps calm the nervous system, the lavender helps quell nausea and ease headache pain, and the rose is a good skin toner. Sunshine dragon marries high-quality Japanese gyokuro with chamomile, marigold, and hints of lemon and orange. The lemon and orange add small amounts of vitamin C, and therefore make this a reasonable tea to take to alleviate cold symptoms. This reviving brew is especially appreciated during the dog days of August. For directions on how to prepare iced green teas, see chapter 7. For information on botanicals other than tea, see chapter 5.

Moroccan mint is probably the most celebrated scented green tea. Rather than using some sort of special mint grown only in Morocco, this tea is prepared by making a bracing infusion of the leaves of spearmint and peppermint sometimes with the addition of other herbs such as absinthium or wild mint. The name refers to more than a type of tea; it describes an entire ceremony of tea taking, which is geared toward caring for the spiritual health of the participants. To learn more about the Moroccan Mint cultural tradition, visit Internet sites such as www.about. com/moroccanfood for a full description. As to physical health, Moroccan mint tea can be viewed as a supreme digestive aid, especially appreciated by those who travel to exotic locations where they may eat unfamiliar food.

Finally, instead of drinking the traditional black earl grey tea described in chapter 2, you may wish to purchase green earl grey tea with its signature bergamot scent. If you cannot find it at the store, try growing your own bergamot and adding it to any green tea. Like most mints, it is easy to cultivate in a wide variety of climates and can even be tended in a flowerpot placed in a sunny window. Add a few fresh leaves to your favorite green brew, steep until you get the flavor you want, and pour over ice.

Four

White Tea

This chapter discusses the health benefits of white tea and describes some types. It is necessarily a short chapter because white tea is a form of green tea, and green tea has already been discussed.

White tea is so named because the silver fuzz that still covers the immature buds and leaves after they are picked turns white when they are dried. As you learned in chapter 1, white tea is a kind of green tea. Therefore, most of the health benefits described in chapter 3 also apply to white tea. However, a few studies have been performed that relate specifically to white tea.

White teas contains a high level of antioxidants because the leaves and buds are steamed and dried immediately after harvesting, locking in their antioxidant qualities.

Because of this kind of processing, white tea contains far less caffeine than other types of tea. Also, as you will discover in chapter 7 on brewing, this type of tea is brewed at a slightly cooler temperature.

Here are some specific health benefits inherent in white tea:

- The polyphenols in white tea can help fight fatigue and wrinkles due to aging. This conclusion is the result of a study done by T. S. A. Thring, P. Hili, and D. P. Naughton at Kingston University in London and published in the *Journal of Inflammation*.

- Because of its high antioxidant content, white tea can help prevent various cancers better than other types of tea by destroying free radicals. The Linus Pauling Institute at Oregon State University in Corvallis conducted a study on mice published in the journal *Carcinogenesis*, using subjects that were genetically predisposed to cancer. The results of this study suggest that white tea can prevent cancerous colon tumors.

- For the same reason, white tea can effectively bolster the body's immune system against a variety of bacteria and diseases. M. Schiffenbauer conducted a study at Pace University on "The Anti-Bacterial, Antifungal, and Anti-Viral Effect of White Tea" that showed how white tea kills Staphylococcus and Streptococcus infections as well as bacteria that cause pneumonia.

- The same study mentioned above suggested that the fluoride in white tea can help prevent tooth decay by slowing the growth of dental plaque.

Types of White Tea

Fewer varieties of white tea exist than green or black teas. As with green tea, white teas are often found scented to add flavor. Fruits make popular additions and health wise, add extra nutrients, specifically vitamin C. Here are some varieties:

- **Silver Needle**—This type of white tea is said to be of the highest quality, and therefore, is the most popular. Ivory colored when dried, this variety is made from exclusively from the buds coming from the Fujian province of China.

- **White Peony**—Is also a popular tea that looks whitish to clear in the cup. The buds and the top leaves are picked before they open and are allowed to wither only slightly. After withering, they are dried by a hot air process that prevents further oxidation and preserves nutrients and freshness. A high-quality white peony will have both the bud and leaf covered in silvery white hair.

- **Long Life Eyebrow**—This tea is concocted from the leaves left over after harvesting for silver needle and white peony. This, however, does not mean that the health benefits are fewer as this tea is processed in much the same way as the other white teas.

- **White Darjeeling**—This type of tea is produced in a similar way to silver needle tea, but because it is grown and processed in the Darjeeling region of India, it tastes more earthy and contains more caffeine and fewer antioxidants.

- **Yin Zhen**—This very slightly oxidized white tea uses only first flush leaf shoots. Yin zhen is the most expensive, but it is famous for its antioxidant and body cooling properties, so it makes a good tea to drink during the hot summer months.

White Tea in Color Healing

Most white teas look yellow to clear in the cup. The yellow hue is a sunny balance between the red and blue ends of the spectrum. The color yellow is linked to creativity, inspiration, mental agility, magnetism, communication, and altruism. Drink yellow-colored teas when you aspire to make a sudden change in your life, achieve success in the performing arts, medicine, diplomacy or counseling, or when you want to charm or persuade. Yellow teas can help you modify your own attitudes, too. Overcome a bad habit, accept a situation you cannot change, and gain the confidence to reach your highest goals with yellow-colored teas. The yellow-colored white teas combine especially well with ginger, both of which are aids to digestion. The vanilla milk tea recipe toward the end of this book in the Recipes section makes use of both white tea and ginger.

White teas can also look clear to whitish in the cup, so in color healing, they also fit the white category. It is difficult to get a tea to look completely white unless you add milk because the nature of tea coloration is to be clear. This color represents clarity, spiritual enlightenment, cleansing, clairvoyance, healing, and truth seeking. As to physical health, white teas are good for detoxification.

Five

Herbal Teas

This chapter details data on herbal teas. It is divided into sections that include: ten important herbal tea ingredients for healthy living; spices to add; three popular herbal teas for better health, which include rooibos, honeybush, and gingko; dandelion root and chicory as coffee substitutes; yerba mate tea; other herbs that can be made into herbal teas and their health benefits; and plants to avoid.

As was explained in chapter 1, herbal teas are not real teas, but many herbs can be brewed and drunk as one might do with tea. These concoctions offer various health benefits. Most herbal teas do not contain any caffeine. Yerba mate is a notable exception.

It is a known fact that humans have drunk herbal teas for pleasure and better health for over two thousand years. However, they have undoubtedly been consumed long before that, probably since some ancient ancestor discovered that fire could boil water. An almost inexhaustible body of knowledge and folk wisdom about herbal teas' healing properties has been amassed over the centuries. More information is being added by both herbalists and scientists every day. As you deepen and broaden your understanding of tea, you may find that others may prefer the taste of herbal brews or that some people may be too caffeine-sensitive to tolerate regular tea. For those readers, this chapter will be doubly informative.

While most edible botanicals contain vitamins, minerals, and antioxidants to fight cancer and other diseases, some contain these elements in more concentrated doses, while others emphasize one or two components to the exclusion of others. Following is a list of ten herbs that can be brewed into teas and consumed for better health. Each botanical works in a different way for healthy living.

If you already are familiar with beverage herbal teas, you will notice that a few popular herbs such as chamomile and peppermint are not included in this initial list. They are discussed later in the chapter. Since they are so well known, it has been decided to offer choices that are equally commendable but not quite as common. You can prepare the following botanicals as singles or blend some together according to your needs and creativity. To add zing and even more therapeutic benefits, you can also add bits of the spices described later in this chapter. Information about an array of botanicals that can be brewed to make herbal teas follows later in the chapter.

Blackberry

Blackberries are not true berries, but rather an aggregate fruit, composed of many little fruits. The trailing variety can be rather a nuisance in the garden, as the vines are prickly and can trip you. However, they do sprout many leaves, which is a good thing when it comes to making blackberry tea, as this is the part used.

Although blackberry fruit contains a lot of natural sugar, both the berries and leaves are nutritious. They contain anthocyanins, folate, vitamins C and K, magnesium, and manganese. Blackberries and blackberry leaf have been proven to reduce cholesterol and flush plaque deposits from the arteries, lessen inflammation, and prevent the free radical damage that can lead to cancer. A study that bears out these claims was published in the *International Journal of Antimicrobial Agents*. The juice and tea made from the leaves are used in folk medicine to treat diarrhea. A traditional remedy for bleeding gums is to chew the leaves.

Borage

Common Names: Bee bread, bugloss, burridge, starflower

This fuzzy-leafed herb with purplish-blue, star-like flowers flourishes in wastelands and multiplies rapidly in the garden. The flowers attract hoards of honeybees, which nowadays with the collapse of so many bee colonies is important to ecology.

In *The Treasurie of Hidden Secrets and Commodious Conceits*, a sixteenth-century English herbal, the anonymous author advises, "The virtue of the conserve of borage is especially good against melancholie; it maketh one merie." Today one might agree that this herb makes a person merry in the sense that the leaves reduce fever, cause urine to flow for those having trouble going to the bathroom, softens and protects the skin, and causes milk to flow in lactating women. Borage tea mixed with lemon, sugar, and perhaps a thimbleful of wine cures a sore throat and restores strength after a long illness. The tea is also good in cases of lung disease that is, according to a study done in the scientific journal *Critical Care Medicine* performed by researchers from the University of Tennessee. Because borage causes perspiration, it helps eliminate toxins from the body. In naturopathic medicine, borage is said to lift the spirits and strengthen resolve.

Calendula
Common Names: Marigold, pot marigold

Besides using the flowers to make tea, the blossoms color cheese, cloth, and hair. They also make an attractive edible garnish. Only the leaves and flowers of the common orange variety possess any medicinal value. The tea strengthens the heart, liver, and kidneys, eases menstrual tension, and expels toxins. Drink the tea as a remedy for headache, toothache, mouth infections, flu, gastric ulcers, red eyes, and jaundice. Since calendula lessens inflammation, you can drink the tea to help eradicate skin problems such as eczema, rashes, dermatitis, and superficial wounds. This is according to an evidence-based systematic review of this botanical performed by E. Basch., S. Bent, and I. Foppa, et al., and published in the *Journal of Herb Pharmacotherapy.* Or make a salve of the flowers and apply it externally to the problem area.

Fennel

Common Name: Sweet fennel

More than three hundred species of this flowering evergreen shrub are known to exist. Fennel is similar to dill and anise in appearance, taste, and therapeutic action. Both the fresh herb and seeds are used to sweeten tea. The taste, though sweet, is strongly licorice-like and very much like anise. If you want to indulge in a cup of fennel tea, herbalists suggest blending it with milder herbs such as chamomile or lemon balm. If you do not have time or opportunity to prepare fennel tea, you can chew on the seeds to suppress your appetite and alleviate heartburn and bloating after a heavy meal.

Like many herbs, fennel expels gas from the stomach and intestines. It contains vitamin C for immune support and potassium and folate to ease cardiovascular and colonic conditions. Among fennel's many medicinal virtues is its use to prevent or diminish muscle spasms, cramps, convulsions, and nervous tension. This herb helps with coughing up phlegm, and causes milk to flow in lactating women. One of fennel's chemical components, anethole, has been proven to reduce inflammation and recurrence of cancer in animals. This is according to studies performed by the American Institute for Cancer Research noted under the references section.

The main reason some people drink fennel tea is to lose weight. The herb and seeds help suppress the appetite, promote the functioning of the body's systems, maintain health, and increase energy. Fennel can be ingested as a preventative when no disease is present to increase flow of urine and stimulate the digestive tract. Weight loss teas and supplements you find on supermarket shelves often contain fennel as one of the ingredients.

On the flipside, fennel may have estrogenic effects that may interfere with the effectiveness of birth control pills, although this has not been proven conclusively. If you are allergic to carrots or celery, you may also be sensitive to this plant.

Hibiscus
Common Names: Karkade, red sorrel, red tea

Do not confuse this last popular name with rooibos, which comes from another plant described later in this chapter.

More than three hundred species exist of this flowering evergreen shrub-like tree. The red or orange petals are the parts usually used to color and flavor tea because the flower is naturally sweet. The petals also comprise the key ingredient of a popular Egyptian refreshment called Karkade. Other parts of the plant can be used in medicinal teas as well. The root soothes the respiratory and digestive systems and the bark is reputed to regulate the menstrual cycle.

Hibiscus flower tea can be taken to support the immune system. If you fall prey to a virus, you can drink the tea to alleviate your cold symptoms because hibiscus dissolves phlegm. The flowers taken in tea lessen inflammation, kill bacteria, increase the body's circulation, and break up obstructions that reduce the body's energy reserves, such as prolonged, low-grade fevers or sluggish digestion. Hibiscus helps a person go to the bathroom and produce a bowel movement. It also promotes the functioning of the body's systems, maintains health, and increases energy. Finally, according to a study performed by D. L. McKay from Tufts University and presented at the American Heart Association annual meeting, drinking just three cups of hibiscus tea per day can lower blood pressure and prevent heart attack and stroke.

Because of its ability to increase flow of urine and stimulate the digestive tract, it seems that hibiscus may interfere with some painkillers by flushing them from the body too quickly. Another caution about hibiscus flower tea is that you should exercise caution when drinking it during pregnancy as it can cause a miscarriage. Since hibiscus flowers are used to color and improve the flavor of many different herbal teas, if you are pregnant the advice is to check the herbal tea's ingredients lists, especially for those herbal teas that turn red or orange in the cup.

Lemon Verbena
Common Names: Herb louisa, van van, verbena

The lemon-scented leaves of this six-foot shrub native to South America make a refreshingly mild, lemon-tasting tea. Drink it either iced or hot. The flavor combines well with mint and stronger-tasting medicinal herbs to help mask their bitterness. The plant is easy to grow and is a perennial in frost-free climates. In cold climates you can substitute hardy lemon balm for lemon verbena. Besides being a tea ingredient, an infusion of the leaves can be applied externally as a wash to clear acne.

Lemon verbena prevents or diminishes muscle spasms, cramps, convulsions, and nervous tension, helps pass gas, promotes sleep, and eases stomachache. Drink the tea also to regulate both diarrhea and constipation. The tea helps lessen nausea and dizziness, combats insomnia, stimulates the brain and improves memory. According to a study performed by N. Caturla, L. Funes, L. Pérez-Fons, and V. Micol and published in the *Journal of Alternative and Complementary Medicine*, this herb can be effectively used to control joint inflammation.

Licorice

Common Name: Sweet root

The origin of the name of this feathery-leafed botanical comes from a Greek word meaning "sweet root." The term is apt because the part of the plant used in medicine and tisane-making is the root, which is fifty times sweeter than sugar.

Besides sweetening ice cream, beer, ale, and bitter-tasting medicines, licorice root can be steeped to make a nutritious tea. Because this herb contains substances similar to adrenal cortical hormones, licorice is administered to treat adrenal problems as well as stress-related disorders that can affect the adrenal glands. The tea is drunk to normalize female hormone balance. Along the same lines, licorice is also posited to promote fertility in both males and females. However, overuse by pregnant women may lead to miscarriage.

This herb is a blood purifier. It quiets coughs, lubricates joints, counteracts pain, and encourages healing of the alimentary canal. It expels mucus from the respiratory tract by promoting coughing. Licorice can be brewed into a tea to alleviate hoarseness and stomach and intestinal pains. In a study presented by T. Sandeep to the National Academy of Sciences, a chemical component of licorice called carbenoxolone may slow the decline of cognitive functions in the elderly. Therefore, licorice may help with loss of memory in Alzheimer's and Parkinson's patients.

Doctors recommend that a person not drink licorice tea for more than two weeks at a time. Drinking too much licorice tea can lead to sodium build-up in the body, which may cause ankles and face to swell and raise blood pressure. The root also interferes with the action of a long list of drugs, including Ace-inhibitors, corticosteroids, insulin, oral contraceptives, laxatives, and even aspirin, among others. When you buy licorice tea, make certain it is comprised of real licorice, and not simply a licorice-flavored preparation.

Red Clover

Common Names: Beebread, cow clover, meadow clover, purple clover, trefoil

The pinkish-purple flower tops are the part used in medicinal and beverage teas. The flavor combines especially well with chamomile. Red clover treats toxicity in blood and prevents or diminishes muscle spasms, cramps, convulsions, and nervous tension. It is beneficial in cases of bronchial congestion, asthma, and whooping cough. In herbal medicine, the tea is sometimes drunk to attenuate cancer symptoms.

The grassy, slightly sweet-tasting flowers are also considered a prime female toner. Red clover contains isoflavones, which change to phytoestrogens (plant-based estrogens) in the body. Therefore, some women drink the tea to relieve symptoms of menopause and Pre-Menstrual Syndrome and to help with weight loss. This research, among other findings, was verified by P. Chedraui, G. San Miguel, L. Hidalgo, et al. in the journal *Gynecology Endocrinology*.

As with all botanicals, there can be side effects to drinking red clover preparations, especially in strong decoctions. The beneficial isoflavones present in the herb may also increase bleeding and slow blood clotting. If you are going to have surgery, it is recommended you stop drinking the tea two weeks prior to your surgery date. For the same reason, red clover interferes with many anti-coagulant medications and even some antibiotics.

Rosehips and Petals
Common Names: Dog rose, Persian rose

Rosehips (the mature seed head) are tangy-sweet and can be nibbled on right off the bush provided it was not sprayed with pesticides. They contain more vitamin C than most botanicals. Unfortunately the vitamin content tends to degrade on drying and during storage. The hips lend a tart, citrus flavor and red color to tea, which is significant in color healing.

In a beverage tea the petals lend a light, delicate aroma. Rosehips, buds, and petals provide such pretty additions to herbal teas that naturopathic healers claim them to be mood elevators that invigorate the heart chakra. This notion is based, in part, on the antioxidant properties of roses, which help reduce stress and stimulate blood circulation. According to a study performed by K. Winther, K. Apel, and G. Thamsborg and published in the *Scandinavian*

Journal of Rheumatolgy, a powder made from the seeds and shells reduces the symptoms of knee and hip osteoarthritis.

Both the petals and hips constrict and bind soft issue and are used to check internal and external secretions like diarrhea and bleeding. They also soothe the pain of stomach ulcers and gallstones. Because of the high vitamin C content, people have been drinking rosehip tea for centuries to help cure colds and flu. At the same time, the vitamin C may interfere with aspirin, estrogen medications, and medicines that keep blood from clotting.

Spearmint
Common Names: Lamb mint, garden mint, spire mint

Many readers will be familiar with the fresh, minty taste of peppermint tea, but perhaps not with its cousin, spearmint. The scent of this wooly mint in the teacup is herbaceous, mellow, and green.

As the common name Lamb Mint implies, spearmint leaves are consumed and the tea is drunk to quell nausea (especially during pregnancy), calm indigestion, and expel gas after eating fatty foods such as lamb. Spearmint helps the stomach produce bile for better digestion; this is the reason some after dinner mints often contain spearmint. Spearmint lessens inflammation of the digestive tract and eases the symptoms of diarrhea and IBS (Irritable Bowel Syndrome). This is according to results of research on the radioprotective potential of mint published by M. S. Baliga and S. Rao in the *Journal of Cancer Research and Therapeutics.*

You can also drink spearmint tea to alleviate cold symptoms such as sore throat and respiratory tract inflammation. The tea also aids oral hygiene as it kills germs in the mouth and lessens toothache pain. Do not drink it too hot or you may irritate the tooth more. Spearmint also contains some vitamin C.

Spices and Other Tea Additives

Next are offered eleven ingredients to spice up your teas for both better health and flavor. You probably already have them in your spice cabinet or can easily obtain them at the supermarket. Each botanical contains antioxidants, vitamins, and minerals. Since you will use mere pinches in your teacup, their beneficial properties will be less evident than those of the tea herbs. Consider them as you might the enhanced RTD waters for sale at the supermarket. Because most either are piquant like cinnamon, have a concentrated flavor like vanilla extract, or taste strong, some people do not like drinking most of them as teas on their own. Ginger, parsley, and sage are exceptions.

Almond Extract

The savory nut of this pink-flowering tree is renowned in culinary circles. Since medieval times, sweet almonds, often simmered in milk, have infused soups and sauces with voluptuous flavor. While the nut is packed with plenty of protein, vitamins, and minerals, the extraction process eliminates all but the taste. Almond extract lends a distinctive fruity note to Mexican hot chocolate, so it also makes a great addition to the chocolate tea described earlier. If you want to reap almond's health benefits, add pieces of the nut to the brew.

Only use extract of sweet almond oil; bitter almond oil contains hydrocyanic acid, a highly volatile and deadly poison. The almond flavoring available at your supermarket is perfectly safe. Even better for your health, you can buy organic extract at most health food groceries. Just make sure not to use a raw source. Frontier Cooperative Herbs makes a delicious organic almond extract, supplied to many chains around the country.

In naturopathic medicine, almonds are deemed to foster harmony and stability in one's life and relationships.

Basil

This bushy annual of the mint family is a familiar sight in many kitchen gardens and windows. The crushed leaves' peppery aroma replicates an intriguing mingling of mint, clove, and anise. Forty basil cultivars exist including lemon, cinnamon, white, purple, and thyme. The most popular is sweet basil.

In herbal medicine, crushed basil leaf infusions are recommended to relieve kidney pain and burning urination. This botanical is also commended as an antioxidant and for its ability to lessen inflammation. Basil tea has been proved to lower bad cholesterol levels and attenuate headaches and fever. It also contains vitamins K and A, magnesium, and manganese. Naturopathic healers believe that basil encourages self-confidence, stability, leadership potential, achievement and mental acuity, and helps regenerate body, mind, and spirit.

If you decide to drink basil tea, tea experts suggest that you combine it with something less pungent, such as green tea, lemon balm, or lemon verbena.

Cardamom

The hot, zesty, reddish-brown seeds of this bushy perennial have traveled over the caravan routes in the Middle East since ancient times. In those days they were mainly used in perfumery. Today cardamom plantations thrive in the West Indies and Central America. The seeds are an acclaimed culinary spice and often are used as a pepper substitute. Cardamom flavors breads, custards, coffee, mulled wine, liqueurs, hot milk, and chai, among other teas.

For centuries, the seeds have been praised as an aphrodisiac and fertility booster, although there is no scientific evidence to the effect. What has been proven is that cardamom contains vitamin C, riboflavin, niacin and B6. This information is according to the USDA SR-21 and reported at www.SelfNutritionData.com. The seeds are also rich in minerals, including calcium, potassium, phosphorus, magnesium, iron, sodium, manganese, and traces of zinc and copper. Cardamom has been prescribed to cure a collection of ailments from dysentery to lung congestion, tooth and gum infections, and more recently,

Celiac disease. It has even been applied externally as an antidote for scorpion and snake bites.

Grind the seeds before adding them to tea. Be careful not to overdo because cardamom is a purgative in large doses.

Cinnamon

Cinnamon is extracted from the inner bark of a medium-sized tropical tree. There are two kinds of cinnamon. Each contains slightly different components, and some gourmands disparage Cassia cinnamon as tasting inferior. True cinnamon, sometimes called "Ceylon cinnamon," in its uncut form looks like one piece of paper rolled into a single spiral, whereas cheap cinnamon is actually bark from the Cassia tree and is identified by its darker color and double-scrolled appearance; i.e., both edges are curled to meet in the middle. Because most frequently you will probably use cinnamon in its powdered form, you will not know how to recognize it by these descriptions and will simply have to read the label, looking for the appropriate Latin name. For the purposes of this manual, if you are not sure which cinnamon to purchase, it is a moot point, for the health benefits of both types are pretty much the same.

Cinnamon is a versatile spice that destroys or prevents bacterial growth, sepsis, and putrefaction. It also is capable of destroying fungus. Herbalists also recommend cinnamon to cure headaches, reduce back pain, flatulence, vomiting, diarrhea, especially from E. coli, and to invigorate memory and cognitive function. There is some scientific evidence that cinnamon reduces the proliferation of leukemia and lymphoma cells. Studies have shown that this spice produces insulin and lowers blood sugar levels for diabetics and LDL (bad) cholesterol levels for the rest of the population. This research was published by T. Lu, H. Sheng, J. Wu, et al. online in the journal *Nutrition Research*. Because cinnamon can stabilize blood sugar levels, and therefore curbs appetite, it has been extolled as a weight loss aid. Chai tea contains some cinnamon and cardamom.

This stimulating bark also enjoys a reputation as an aphrodisiac. At the same time, the spice imparts energy of a peaceful nature. Although cinnamon tea recipes exist, drinking pure cinnamon tea is not recommended because its intense spiciness can burn the mouth. Sprinkle just a few granules in everyone's tea to foster a happy, harmonious home environment.

The disadvantage to cinnamon is that an overdose can interfere with a range of diabetes medications. Taken in large amounts, it can also irritate the liver. Then again, since everything people consume is processed by the liver, doses of any quantity can affect it. More to the point, because essential oil of cinnamon can burn the skin and cause severe eye irritation, herbalists recommend that you handle both the oil and powder with care.

Citrus Peels and Juice

Chapter 2 described how citrus peels add gusto to Constant Comment black tea. If used judiciously, they can work the same miracle on herbal teas, especially those infusions and decoctions with bitter-tasting ingredients.

Lemon juice can infuse vitality into many kinds of tea. Since lemons are sour, the recommendation is to add only a squirt or two. Use the peel instead, and you get the punch without the pucker. When buying lemons for the peel or juice, avoid those with coarse, deep yellow-colored skin, as they tend to yield less juice and the peel tastes grainy. Lightly roll the fruit between your thumb and forefinger to estimate its juiciness. The same applies to limes.

Lemons are a superb blood purifier also known to promote urination as well as the functioning of the body's systems. Lemons help maintain physical health and increase energy. They can be ingested as a preventative when no disease is present. They can also increase the body's circulation and break up obstructions that reduce the body's energy reserves, such as prolonged low-grade fevers or sluggish digestion. Be careful not to drink lemon in too concentrated a dose as the acid can damage tooth enamel. This remarkable fruit is said to refresh and stimulate the mind, but also relax nervous, overly talkative people. If you want to get your point across at the dinner table without constant interruptions, serve iced lemon tea.

As orange juice companies let everyone know in their advertisements, this fruit is an excellent source of vitamin

C and calcium. Oranges, including the peel, also contain a fair portion of thiamine, a B vitamin that helps deliver oxygen to the body; folic acid, which is important for fetal brain development; and potassium, an important mineral to help the body achieve electrolyte balance. The antioxidants in oranges are purported to alleviate symptoms of rheumatism, pneumonia, and arthritis, and help alcoholics resist cravings. Just sniffing the sweet fragrance of grated orange zest is believed to counteract depression, insomnia, premenstrual syndrome, hysteria, and a range of psychosomatic illnesses. If you are fortunate enough to live in a citrus-growing region, you can pluck your own orange blossoms and infuse them into any tea to cleanse your digestive system.

Clove

The piquant essence of clove is extracted from the unopened buds of an aromatic evergreen cultivated in the East and West Indies, Ceylon, Mauritius, Brazil, Guinea, and Sumatra. A term for clove in some Middle Eastern countries is "nail," and indeed the buds look like miniature nails.

During the devastating plagues that hit Medieval Europe, clove essence was applied to sponges and handkerchiefs as a purifying agent. Modern science has since discovered that clove oil kills typhoid germs and fungus and destroys or prevents bacterial growth, sepsis, and putrefaction. Among other studies that corroborate this statement is one that was performed at the Universidade Metolodistsa de Piracicaba, São Paulo, Brazil and reported in the *Brazilian Journal of Microbiology*. English smelling salts rely on a mixture of cloves, cinnamon, lavender, camphor, and aniseed. If you eliminate the camphor, which is poisonous if swallowed, you can make an energizing herbal tea from the other ingredients.

For centuries, toothache sufferers have applied oil of clove to their gums to deaden the pain while waiting to see the dentist. Put bruised clove buds into your tea to release the painkilling essence and accomplish the same task. Clove also helps quell stomach gases and eliminates bad breath.

Eugenol, one of clove's chemical constituents, slows blood clotting, so it tends to magnify the effects of blood thinners. Therefore, clove tea is not recommended during pregnancy because it may cause miscarriage. On the other hand, when a woman is about to give birth, drinking a cup of clove tea may strengthen uterine contractions and help ease delivery. This tea is not recommended for children as it can cause liver damage and, rarely, seizures.

Clove buds will improve the taste of most medicinal infusions and decoctions. As with cinnamon, you will want to add them in small doses. Nonetheless, some people enjoy drinking pure clove tea. If you wish to experiment, herbalists suggest that you buy whole cloves as the powdered spice loses much of its strength in storage. Test the buds for freshness by pinching one between your thumb and forefinger to release the oil.

Ginger

Ginger, a tropical perennial with a knobby, aromatic root-stalk, is a versatile culinary ingredient used in pies, cakes, biscuits, cookies, fruit, sauces, bread, meat, and fish. Ginger beer and ginger wine are also enjoyable. Besides drinking ginger tea, some people like to take ginger in homemade, carbonated ginger lemonade. Ginger and lemon taste especially good combined in a tea, and many tea companies offer ginger and lemon teabags.

This stimulating rhizome (underground rootstalk) is beneficial for flatulent colic, diarrhea, kidney trouble, and chest complaints. The polyphenols in ginger help overcome motion sickness and nausea experienced after operations and chemotherapy. For more than two-thousand years, people have consumed ginger tea to alleviate symptoms of coughs and colds. Ginger can also motivate the metabolism when dieting. Use the powder or boil clean, chopped fresh pieces of the rhizome and siphon off the liquid for a tisane. In naturopathic medicine, ginger is a reputed aphrodisiac and considered to be a remedy for frigidity.

Ginger is a fairly safe herb, but since it tends to lower blood pressure, it may increase the effects of high blood pressure medications. Because it lessens inflammation, it also may interfere with blood thinners and diabetes medicines. Drinking too much ginger tea can also irritate the lining of the inside of the mouth and cause heartburn.

Parsley

Undoubtedly you recognize the lacy green leaves of this ubiquitous biennial kitchen herb as a garnish. However, you may be surprised to learn that parsley also makes a healthful, refreshing, and delicious addition to herbal teas. The curly-leaf variety is more popular, but flat-leafed parsley has a stronger taste. When you bring a bunch of parsley home from the grocery, be sure to rinse and squeeze it dry to remove clinging dirt. Better yet, grow your own in a kitchen window box. This herb even prefers partial shade, so it can thrive indoors. See chapter 8 for tips on growing herbs indoors.

People used to believe that parsley increased vitality and strength. This is one reason it was twisted into wreaths to crown victors at the ancient Olympic games. Perhaps here is an instance of a coincidental relationship between fact and fancy. Scientists have since found parsley to be rich in vitamins A, B_1, B_2, B_3, and C, as well as iron, potassium, and fiber, all of which increase vitality. This garnish stimulates the appetite, increases urine flow, is a reliable digestive, and minimizes intestinal gas. Parsley is said to be a great cleanser and would be an excellent detox tea.

Parsley tea is sometimes drunk to bring on a woman's period because it encourages blood to flow toward the uterus and cervix. Because of this action, parsley tea can also cause miscarriage. The herb also contains high amounts of oxalic acid, so it can stimulate formation of kidney stones, exacerbate symptoms of kidney and liver disease, and even cause balance problems. The key to drinking parsley tea, therefore, is moderation. Pinches of it, together with other herbs in a tea, are not likely to have a deleterious effect. The leaf, seeds, and root are all used medicinally, but the fresh chopped or dried leaf is drunk mainly as an herbal tea.

Sage

This evergreen of the mint family is native to the Mediterranean. The grayish-green leaves are the part used in herbal tea-making. Of the many types, the wild variety imparts a fresh herbal scent to High Country meadows, especially after a cooling rain. Many sage varietals exist, and many plants are called "sage," but not all are related to the plant. Unrelated plants can be used in incense making, potpourri, and sachets, but for the most part they do not substitute well in herbal teas and do not carry the same nutrients.

Sage leaves prevent or diminish muscle spasms, cramps, convulsions, and nervous tension, decrease or prevent fever, destroy or prevent bacterial growth, sepsis, and putrefaction, and help pass gas. Along with yarrow, which also tends to grow in meadows, the leaves of this were applied to open wounds incurred on the battlefield in times gone by. The herbal tea and extract of the leaves are sometimes taken to promote conception. However, once the pregnancy is established, one should avoid drinking sage tea because it can also bring on a miscarriage.

Clary sage, a related plant, strengthens the eyes, stomach, uterus, kidneys, and back. Naturopathic healers believe it is a good herbal tea for anyone engaged in creative pursuits. However, epileptics should stay away from it, and especially avoid using the essential oil because it exercises a strong effect on the central nervous system.

Prevent a cold by preparing an herbal tea from sage leaves, lemon, and honey. This tea is also recommended to ease the soreness of tonsillitis. An infusion of sage leaves will slow the flow of bodily excretions such as night sweats, postnasal drip, and external bleeding. Sage tea can also eliminate canker sores and nervous headaches and purify the liver and kidneys. The flavor of the leaves combines especially well with those of mint and rosemary and will add the nutritive benefits of those botanicals to the brew.

Thyme

Although this herb has a balsamic odor, the pungent taste can overwhelm a tea. Nonetheless, it is often recommended as a medicinal and beverage tea ingredient. Folk healers of old were empiricists, and through observation and experimentation, they learned to value thyme as one of the essential botanicals of the herbal pharmacopeia. Modern science has corroborated their findings. According to the website www.nutrition-and-you.com where nutrients of various botanicals are measured and published, a mere 100 grams of fresh thyme leaves provide the following percentages of the recommended daily allowance for adults of vitamins and minerals:

- 150% of vitamin A

- 27% of vitamin B_6 (pyridoxine)

- 266% of vitamin C

- 40% of calcium

- 38% of dietary fiber

- 218% of iron

- 40% of magnesium

- 75% of manganese

The leaves, the part used to brew an herbal tea, destroy or prevent bacterial growth, sepsis, and putrefaction. The study cited above for cloves also mentions this benefit for thyme. Thyme prevents or diminishes muscle spasms, cramps, convulsions, and nervous tension, helps pass gas, and expels mucus from the respiratory tract by promoting coughing. Those same folk healers spoken of earlier have been using thyme in conjunction with plantain to cure these aliments for centuries. The tea is drunk along with other ingredients to ease symptoms of sinusitis and flu.

When you brew thyme, be sure to cover it while it steeps. You do not want to lose any of those precious vitamins, minerals, and essential oils to evaporation.

Vanilla Extract

The pod (called a bean) of this creeping, greenish-yellow orchid native to Mexico and Central America sweetens all kinds of dishes, including cookies, cakes, custards, and sugar as well as liqueurs. Though they are expensive, you can reuse a vanilla bean many times in cooking as long as you wash and dry it.

Vanilla essence increases the body's circulation and breaks up obstructions that reduce the body's energy reserves, such as prolonged, low-grade fevers or sluggish digestion. It also has been hailed as a sexual stimulant since the time of the Maya, but there is no scientific evidence to support this claim. What has been verified is that vanilla's chemical components produce a calming effect. It can be added to teas to soothe emotional trauma and gain tranquility and peace of mind. Naturopathic healers recommend this tenacious essence to stimulate the mind, and promote endurance, inspiration, intuition, patience, and facilitate better organizational skills. Vanilla beans also contain some B-complex vitamins to regulate the metabolism and nervous system.

Traces of various minerals are also present, namely potassium, copper, and manganese. A study performed by the Central Food Technological Institute in Mysore, India has shown that the antioxidants in vanilla reduce the proliferation of free radicals. The extract has also been shown to help regulate the menstrual cycle. The scent of vanilla in tea can help with weight loss because it tastes sweet and filling.

The most convenient way to use vanilla in tea is to add a few drops of the extract to your brew. The extract is prepared by boiling the bean with alcohol and water, although a few companies produce the extract without the alcohol. The result is a concentrated vanilla flavor.

Vanilla mates best with black tea. The fragrance and taste also meld deliciously with almond extract, blueberry, clove, cranberry, honey, honeybush, and pomegranate.

Although vanilla is considered a safe product, you need to be careful to buy pure vanilla bean extract. Because it is so expensive (only saffron is more pricey), some companies dilute their vanilla with cheaper extracts. Worse, some, although not all, Mexican vanilla extracts are made from a combination of vanilla and coumarin. Coumarin, which smells exactly like vanilla, is poisonous if eaten. It has been banned for use in food by the FDA since the 1950s.

The next section of this chapter focuses on the health benefits to be derived from drinking teas concocted from three especially popular botanicals, rooibos, honeybush, and gingko.

Rooibos and Honeybush

Rooibos and honeybush herbal teas are often considered identical because they hail from the same corner of the world. Certainly, both bushes look red in the teacup and they share many healing traits. Nonetheless, they are two distinct plants.

Rooibos

Rooibos, also known as the six-foot red bush shrub, grows only in the rugged mountains of the Cedarberg district of South Africa, 175 kilometers north of Cape Town. The indigenous population introduced this tea to Dutch settlers and showed them how to process it in much the same way as black tea. The leaves were chopped, bruised, raked into piles to oxidize in the strong African sun, and then dried. The Dutch fell in love with the processed leaves' slightly sweet, tobacco-like taste and rich, mahogany hue. The pennywise Dutch were also quick to recognize that rooibos cost little compared to high-priced imported tea.

Although people knew about rooibos, it was difficult to obtain it outside of South Africa until cultivation was finally commercialized in the 1930s. It was not until the 1980s, when earlier research into the leaves' medicinal components finally came to light, that rooibos caught the public eye. The world has the Japanese to thank for popularizing this herbal infusion because of their belief in its antiaging properties. Anything that promises to slow aging also makes a big splash in American, youth-oriented society.

Research has shown that rooibos is the only known source of aspalathin, an antioxidant with the capacity to reverse the progress of skin cancer and other dermatological diseases. (Source: *Nutrition Research,* 2008, Oct. 28.) This chemical is also responsible for healing respiratory, allergic, and digestive conditions as well as diabetes and heart problems. Rooibos contains a high concentration of vitamin C, calcium, zinc and alpha-hydroxy acid, which stimulates hair growth and skin cell renewal. Some health professionals are hopeful that this botanical may help cure HIV as well, but more research in this area needs to be done.

There is another reason rooibos and honeybush are linked besides those mentioned above. When consumed together in an infusion, they eliminate cancerous skin tumors entirely and keep them from recurring, at least in mice.

Rooibos' dark red color emerges when the leaves are fully oxidized. If instead they are dried quickly without any oxidation like green tea, the leaves stay green. There is a distinct difference in flavor, however, as much of the sweetness comes about with oxidation. To overcome the more bitter taste of the green rooibos, commercial tea companies often blend it in teabags together with berries, caramel, mango, or mint.

Honeybush

Honeybush is an entire species of bushes also native to South Africa. The bushes grow along the coast in the region just south of Cedarberg. Some species thrive in the mountains, but others are harvested on wet southern slopes, marshy areas, and in hilly streambeds. Honeybush is not cultivated, so the harvesting is done by gathering from natural populations. This makes for an uneven quality.

Some enthusiasts maintain that this unrefined, organic harvesting method adds value to the medicinal virtues of the tea while others remain skeptical.

While rooibos infusions are brewed exclusively from leaves, the gorgeous yellow flowers, sweetly scented leaves, and softer stems go into making honeybush tea. The best quality material is found on young bushes. Many bushes are severely pruned so that newer shoots can be harvested the following season. Harvesting of a single bush occurs every two to three years.

The organic materials are fermented either in the traditional way in piles, or cured in a low-heat oven until the green color changes to dark brown and exudes a sweet, honey-like scent. Oven oxidation results in a more standardized product, but the dried materials are not as attractive as when the traditional method is used. After fermentation, the tea is dried and ready to drink.

Like rooibos, honeybush is caffeine- and pesticide-free and its tannic content is low. The herbal infusion is mineral-rich, including calcium, copper, iron, magnesium, manganese, potassium, sodium, and zinc. It also contains substantial amounts of the chemical Pinitol, which helps expel mucus from the respiratory tract by promoting coughing.

Honeybush is loaded with flavones, isoflavones and xanthines, antioxidants that combat viruses, fungi, and microbes that invade the body. Honeybush tea can ease digestive problems; bolster the immune system; shrink allergic reactions; battle free radicals; reduce the risk of osteoporosis, breast, uterine, and prostate cancer; lower cholesterol levels; and regulate the menstrual cycle. Currently studies are being conducted to determine whether the plant inhibits fat accumulation in the body and helps break down existing fat cells. (Source: article published in the journal *Phytomedicine* by D. Zulfagar, J. Louw, C. Muller, et al.) If this turns out to be true, honeybush may rocket to stardom as a miracle weight-loss supplement.

To derive the most therapeutic benefits from the tea, it seems more effective to take it together with rooibos. This makes sense, since the two types of bushes are such good neighbors. Besides, the two teas taste better together. Honeybush is more full-bodied and sweeter. The taste has been described as something between hot apricot jam, dried fruit, and honey.

Gingko

Gingko, sometimes spelled "ginkgo" and "ginko," and also known as *Gingko biloba*, is a tree. It is often referred to as the "fossil tree" because it is the oldest living tree on record, dating back to before the time of the dinosaurs. A single specimen can soar to 120 feet and live for a thousand years. Although it is native to China, gingko has been planted as an ornamental worldwide. The leaves are the part used in herbal medicine. They have two lobes and a fanlike shape that makes them look like a maidenhair fern; this is the reason it is often called the "maidenhair tree."

Although gingko is relatively new to Western herbalism, it has been used in Chinese medicine for more than two thousand years as a remedy for multiple ailments such as the dizziness, headache, and fatigue brought on by altitude sickness as well as memory loss in old age. Due to the interest researchers are taking in this botanical as a possible cure for Alzheimer's and other cognitive disorders, gingko has soared to the top of the list of fast-selling herbal supplements. The tea has been proven, among other studies, by research conducted at the University of Maryland Medical Center and published in the *Cochrane Database Systems Review* to aid cognitive speed and prevent the progression of dementia resulting from atherosclerotic vascular disease.

Its anticoagulant properties help with circulatory problems, principally leg pain, and improve blood flow. This benefit, in turn, helps relieve symptoms of pre-menstrual syndrome and age-related eye disorders like cataracts, glaucoma, and macular degeneration. Research is being carried out, but has not yet been completed, on its effectiveness in treating ringing in the ears, depression, attention deficit, multiple sclerosis, and other autoimmune and psychological disorders.

Certain risks are involved with drinking a gingko infusion. Although it is generally safe, gingko causes blood to flow. If you suffer from a bleeding disorder or are on blood thinners, you should talk to your doctor about its safety. For some sensitive people, gingko can cause dizziness, headache, diarrhea, nausea, gas, and heart palpitations. Under no circumstances should you drink tea made from the raw plant materials. Uncooked gingko seeds, if consumed, can cause seizure and death.

It seems that even a medicinal strength preparation of the tea is not as potent as the supplements. If you are looking for fast, definitive relief from the above-listed symptoms, herbalists recommend you opt for the pills. As to gingko's taste, some claim that it is delicate and sweet; others complain about the woody, bark-like flavor.

Health Benefits of Botanical Coffee Substitutes

The next section of this chapter discusses the health benefits of botanicals that can be drunk in herbal teas as coffee substitutes. These include chicory, dandelion root, and yerba mate, a botanical that does not taste like coffee, but which does contain a lot of caffeine.

Chicory

Up to now, this book has focused on an audience of presumed tea drinkers. Perhaps you are a coffee drinker who, for whatever reason, has given up coffee, yet misses the aroma and taste. Or maybe you know someone who feels that way. For those people, chicory may be the answer.

The herb chicory, also known as blue-sailors, coffee weed, and succory makes a credible coffee substitute. During the American Civil War, when the Union cut off the coffee supply to the Confederates, people in the South substituted chicory. Southerners relished the taste so much that today they still enjoy drinking chicory blended with coffee. The New Orleans brand Luzianne, a popular tea company, has a coffee line that includes chicory. The combination of coffee and chicory creates a mellow, aromatic flavor, while reducing the caffeine content by half.

Chicory's long, caffeine-free taproot, which thrives in calcareous conditions hostile to less hardy plants, is the part harvested, chopped, and roasted. In herbal medicine, the root is prescribed to cause urine to flow, produce a bowel movement, detoxify the liver, promote the functioning of the body's systems, maintain health, and increase energy. It can be ingested as a preventative when no disease is present. A poultice fashioned from the crushed root reduces inflammations. It is also used by herbalists to stimulate the intuitive faculties, although there is no scientific evidence to support this claim.

Dandelion

It is said that roasted dandelion root also makes a reasonable alternative to coffee. You can dig, clean, cut, roast, and grind the roots yourself, but the procedure may prove more trouble than it is worth. Besides the time-consuming preparation, you need to verify that the dandelions you dig have not been sprayed with pesticides or chemical fertilizers. People may think they can go to the local playground and pick some dandelions, but this is not always the case! This is also the recommendation for all botanicals gathered in the wild. You can always go the organic commercial route, too. Commercially prepared roasted and powdered dandelion root looks and smells like coffee, and has a similar taste. Look for it at health food stores.

As with chicory, dandelion leaves are a valuable asset in herbal medicine and can be prepared as an herbal tea. However, the leaves taste different from the root.

Dandelion root helps cure urinary, bladder, and kidney infections because it encourages urine to flow. It aids in dissolving kidney stones and flushes toxins from the bladder by lessening fluid retention. The tea also prevents signs of indigestion like heartburn, gas, and bloating. According to studies performed at the University of Maryland Medical Center in 2009 and published in the *American Journal of Clinical Nutrition*, this is due to the fact that the root increases healthy bacteria in the digestive tract. The root contains significant amounts of vitamins C and B, as well as iron, magnesium, potassium, and zinc.

As to the leaves, they are so rich in vitamin C that in former times, dandelion leaf tea was drunk to avert scurvy. The vitamin C content can also be effective in cases of eczema. Perhaps because dandelion heads look so ebullient nodding in the sunshine, naturopathic healers use the plant to help a person overcome emotional trauma.

Mate

Also known as *yerba mate* (pronounced "yer-bah mah-tay" (maté with the accent on the "e" is an affectation), this botanical infusion is not a proper tea because it does not come from the *Camellia sinensis* bush. Mate is gaining popularity, both because of its unique flavor and health benefits. Mate is made from the leaves of a native subtropical South American evergreen, and historically is drunk in Paraguay, Argentina, Brazil, and Uruguay.

Unlike most herbs, mate contains caffeine—a whopping 150 mg per cup, even more than coffee. On the plus side, this means that drinking this herbal tea can increase physical endurance, help enhance the ability to focus, and stimulate digestion. The leaves from the shrub are rich in antioxidants, too, which can support the immune system and protect against multiplication of free radicals in the body. The antioxidants, along with some of the amino acids present in mate, also help flush out fat and bad LDL cholesterol.

On the negative side, because of the high caffeine content, consumption of large amounts of mate over prolonged periods can open the door to certain cancers, including cancer of the mouth, esophagus, lungs, kidneys, and bladder. The caffeine can also cause nervousness, increased and irregular heartbeat, high blood pressure, insomnia, and ringing in the ears for caffeine-sensitive people.

Botanical Infusion Ingredients from Alfalfa to Yerba Santa

This section describes an array of botanicals commonly used to make herbal infusions and decoctions. The botanical and its therapeutic benefits, side effects or precautions, if any, are described. Many botanicals do not have much flavor to them; if they do, it is noted. The end of the chapter lists botanicals to avoid. It is not an all-encompassing list, but most dangerous plants are included.

Alfalfa Leaf

Common Names: Buffalo herb, Chilean clover, lucerne, purple medic

Known to the ancient Arabs as "father of all foods," this grassy perennial is a ready source of minerals such as potassium, magnesium, phosphorous, and calcium; vitamins A, B, C, and K; organic salts; and essential enzymes. The leaves and seeds are the parts used to prepare herbal infusions. Alfalfa's attributes include its use as a nutritive substance to promote the functioning of the body's systems, maintain health, and increase energy. It can be ingested as a preventative when no disease is present to hasten recovery from an illness and for weight loss. Down this infusion to decrease fevers, cure infections, arrest hemorrhages, manage fatigue, alleviate arthritis and asthma symptoms, and lower blood pressure. The light-colored grass looks similar to white tea in the cup, and so can be considered in the same ways as a white tea in color healing. The flavor is bland like grass, or at best, like freshly mown hay. Blending alfalfa with lemon balm, lemon verbena, red clover, or mint will enliven your brew.

Althea Root

Common Names: Marshmallow, mortification root, sweet-
weed

The soft, downy, petiole leaves of this marsh plant
grow on three- to four-foot stems in damp meadows and
ditches. The mucilage made from the root decreases inflammation and soothes the skin. Taken internally as a
tea, althea root placates sore throats and mucus membranes and alleviates signs of constipation and irritable
bowel syndrome. If you have low blood pressure, althea
root may exacerbate the condition, so check with a doctor
before drinking the herbal infusion.

Angelica

Common Names: Archangel, masterwort, root of the
holy ghost, St. Michael's plant

Angelica is a fragrant, leafy plant of the carrot family
that flourishes in cool climates as far north as Iceland and
Lapland. Use the roots, leaves, and seeds to make herbal
beverage teas and medicinal infusions and decoctions. The
seeds scatter everywhere, and before you know it, you will
be rewarded with many seedlings from a single plant. As a
drink, however, angelica's flavor is like celery. It tastes better if you squirt some lemon into the cup as well.

As a healthy tea ingredient, angelica has many uses.
It is a substance that purifies the blood and removes toxins from the circulation, expels gas from the stomach and
intestines, produces perspiration in order to bring down a

fever, causes urine to flow, induces and increases menstrual flow, expels mucus from the respiratory tract by promoting coughing, and breaks up obstructions that reduce the body's energy reserves, such as prolonged low-grade fevers or sluggish digestion. It is considered a tonic to strengthen and tone the stomach and aid digestion. An infusion of the seeds relieves flatulence. It can be ingested as a preventative when no disease is present, combats nausea, and helps cure coughs, colds, pleurisy, colic, and urinary tract infections.

Anise

Common Names: Aniseed, sweet cumin

An umbelliferous annual of the carrot family, anise and fennel look and taste very much alike. Like fennel, anise helps with bloating, bad breath, and nausea. It quiets the digestion and is useful in cases of asthma and colic. Although both anise and fennel make excellent teas, you probably would prefer to brew them in combination with other herbs and not drink the strong-tasting herbs singly as you might do with peppermint or lemon balm leaves. Another choice is to brew the seeds in milk and drink before going to bed to ease digestion and get a good night's sleep.

Anise also expels mucus from the respiratory tract by promoting coughing, relieves gas pains, causes urine to flow, and helps ease digestion of pork and beef. It also contains properties that break up mucus in pectoral infections and soothe hard, dry coughs.

Bergamot

Common Names: Bee balm, oswego tea

This citrusy tasting mint with a touch of pepper is easy to grow and tolerates a wide range of garden conditions. Another plant with the same flavor is also called bergamot and marks the signature flavor of Earl Grey tea. You can add a few fresh bergamot leaves to China Black or Darjeeling tea to replicate the Earl Grey taste.

Drink an infusion to alleviate pain from cancer of the uterus, tumors, and intestinal cramping from premenstrual syndrome or intestinal disorders. The tea also helps in cases of fluid retention, fever, and spasms. Bergamot is drunk to chase away depression. Naturopaths suggest adding it to *Camellia sinensis* tea to spur motivation. Add the infusion to your bath water to help alleviate joints painfully swollen from arthritis. The FDA considers this herb unsafe to use during pregnancy.

Blessed Thistle

Common Names: Holy thistle, spotted thistle

This botanical is so-called because during the Middle Ages it was thought to cure smallpox and other "spotty" diseases. An annual thistle with a hairy brown stem, it grows in wastelands and on roadsides. The spry, yellow flowers bloom on two-foot hairy brown stems from May to August.

The flowering tops, leaves, and upper stems of this botanical are used to alter the condition of a disease by curing the infection. The tea can also be taken in cases of arthritis, cancer, and skin eruptions. The tea produces sweating, increases milk production in lactating women, and brings on a woman's period. Medical experts disagree about this herb's use to increase milk production in lactating women and some warn against drinking the infusion during and after pregnancy. The herbal infusion also combats bacteria.

Some herbalists tout this plant as a natural contraceptive, but there is no scientific evidence to the effect. If you are allergic to artichokes or plants of the Aster family such as marigolds, ragweed, or daisies, you may also be sensitive to this herb. Those suffering from Crohn's disease or intestinal troubles may have their problems exacerbated by drinking the infusion.

Blueberry Leaf
Common Names: Highbush blueberry, lowbush blueberry, American blueberry

Blueberry leaf possesses many of the same medicinal qualities as the fruit. In fact, the leaf contains more antioxidants than the fruit. Basically, blueberry leaf constricts and binds soft tissue to check internal and external secretions like diarrhea and bleeding, acts as a blood purifier and circulation toner, promotes the functioning of the body's systems, maintains health, and increases energy. The tea can be ingested as a preventative when no disease is present after a miscarriage. Both the leaves and fruit are used to prevent cataracts and glaucoma.

Blueberry leaf's hypoglycemic properties have been proven to lower blood sugar levels in diabetics by up to 25 percent. Drink the tea to relieve diarrhea, sore throat, and urinary tract infections. According to WebMD .com, the antioxidants present in blueberry leaves "may help to promote a long-lasting and healthy brain."

Caraway
Common Name: Kummel

Caraway is a common culinary biennial herb of the carrot family similar to anise, dill, and fennel. The plant grows two feet high and has white or yellow flowers and feathery, dusty green or turquoise leaves. The long, tapered root often is confused with deadly water hemlock. Since Roman times, caraway has been used to flavor cookies, bread, cake, soup, cabbage, cheese, and Kummel liqueur.

The herb guards against spasms and is a mild digestive that increases the body's circulation and breaks up obstructions that reduce the body's energy reserves, such as prolonged, low-grade fevers or sluggish digestion. Caraway also helps eliminate intestinal gas and heartburn. This botanical can also increase milk production in lactating mothers. Since the taste of the ground seed in a tea is warm and biting similar to anise and fennel, herbalists recommend adding it sparingly to beverage blends.

Catnip

Common Names: Cat mint, cat's-play

A strong-smelling botanical of the mint family, catnip grows easily in poor soil, and like most mints, spreads rapidly. The white to pinkish flowers form tubular clusters atop square, branching stems. Cats love catnip.

The leaves of this three-foot tall herb are the part used to make the aromatic, minty tea. They prevent or diminish muscle spasms, cramps, convulsions, and nervous tension. Catnip can expel gas from the stomach and intestines and promote sweating in order to bring down a fever or to remove toxins from the body. The tea can calm the central nervous system, promote the functioning of the body's systems, maintain health, and increase energy. Catnip can be ingested as a preventative when no disease is present. It is a slight inducer of a woman's period. Catnip makes an excellent tea for nervous headaches and also helps cure children's diarrhea and general fussiness. Combined in an infusion with lemon balm, althea root, and licorice, it is good for baby's colic, irritability, and colds. If you are not fond of the taste of this particular mint, try lemon-flavored catnip tea, available from many suppliers like the San Francisco Herb Company, or combine it with lemon verbena or lemon balm for a lemony taste.

Cat's Claw
Common Name: Uña de Gato (Spanish)

As its common name attests, cat's claw hails from tropical regions of South America. The bark and root are the parts used to prepare medicinal teas. Cat's claw is principally taken to alleviate symptoms of both rheumatoid and osteoarthritis. Those suffering from intestinal disorders such as diverticulitis and gastritis may find relief using this herb because it cleans out the intestinal tract. It also helps balance hormones. Cat's claw invigorates the immune system. If you suffer from an autoimmune disease such as lupus or multiple sclerosis or have severe allergies, speak to your healthcare professional before starting a regimen.

Chamomile
The name comes from German and means "earth apple." The daisy-like flower of this bright, sturdy little herb is the part used to make infusions. The cheerful-looking flowers fulfill the functions of yellow-colored liquids in color therapy.

Chamomile is also good for the digestion, which will help you sleep well, too, as it is purported to heal during the night. Drink an infusion to ease the pain of menstrual cramps or any gastrointestinal trouble. Chamomile also possesses strong anti-inflammatory properties. Lactating mothers drink the brew to help increase milk production and give it to their children to stop bedwetting. The pleasant, apple-scented flavor of the herbal tea also helps bring

peace of mind as chamomile is the quintessential preparation designed to release nervous tension and irritability
and nourish the nervous system. If you suffer from an allergy to ragweed, you may also be allergic to chamomile,
and therefore should not drink this herbal tea.

Cherry

Besides tasting sweet, the fruit cause urine to flow more
easily and helps improve the eyesight. Cherries are also
an agent that constricts and binds soft tissue to check internal and external secretions like diarrhea and bleeding.
Because they are so sweet but also tangy, a couple of dried
cherries in the cup will perk up any tea or herbal infusion.

Cranesbill

Common Names: Alumroot, wild geranium

This is not the popular potted flower but a wild plant
with pinkish-purplish five-petaled flowers that bloom in
clusters at the end of each stem. A native of North America, cranesbill thrives in the woods in the eastern part of
the United States. The leaves lend an exotic flavor to tea
and combine well with blackberries, blueberries, lemon,
and rose petals. The flowers, which are also edible, can be
added to herbal infusions.

Native North Americans once relied on this herb as a
method of birth control. According to naturopathic practitioners, a cranesbill decoction reduces yin/yang extremes,
calms the nerves, and aids the transition through menopause.

You will often see cranesbill advertised in gardening cata-
logues under the sobriquet "the mosquito repellant plant,"
as it effectively repels mosquitoes and other bothersome
insects. The powdered rhizome is taken in a decoction to
stop diarrhea.

Damiana

Damiana is a somewhat bitter-tasting botanical that grows
as a shrub in the warmer climates of the Western hemi-
sphere. The pale green, ribbed leaves with somewhat hairy
undersides are the part used to prepare herbal teas.

For centuries, herbalists have prescribed drinking damiana tea as a love potion. Modern science has since vali-
dated this herb to be a sexual enhancer for men as well as
an aid for prostate disorders. Damiana also increases the
body's circulation and breaks up obstructions that reduce
the body's energy reserves, such as prolonged, low-grade
fevers or sluggish digestion. This botanical is sometimes
prescribed to women to balance their hormones, increase
fertility, and manage premenstrual syndrome. Damiana
leaf increases urine, makes a person vomit, promotes
the functioning of the body's systems, maintains health,
and increases energy. It can be ingested as a preventative
when no disease is present, and is especially good for the
reproductive system.

Dong Quai

Dong quai is a perennial of the celery family. The plant has smooth purple stems and umbrella-like clusters of fragrant white flowers that look similar to a celery plant gone to seed. However, the root is the part used to make herbal teas. Often it is decocted in wine, sliced and candied or used in extract form.

This is a prime go-to herb for women's disorders. It has been used in Asian or Eastern medicine for more than a thousand years to tone the uterus, stimulate blood flow, correct hormonal imbalances, especially during and after menopause, regulate menses, and stimulate uterine contractions during childbirth. The infusion is also drunk to alleviate nasal congestion, especially stuffiness stemming from allergies.

Be advised that this plant can make a person photosensitive, so it is advisable to stay out of the sun while on a dong quai regimen. Since it causes bleeding, you should not take it if you are on blood thinners.

Echinacea

Common Names: Coneflower, purple coneflower, black sampson

This two-foot-tall herb with the large, pale purple, daisy-like flowers grows wild in the foothills of the Rocky Mountains and on the prairie. Over the last decade, it has become popular as a cold and flu preventative and remedy. Enthusiasts point to the root's (the part used in tea) properties to combat viral and bacterial infections as well as to stimulate the immune system and shorten the length of a cold. This claim has been verified by a study performed by the University of Maryland Medical Center. The herbal infusion is also drunk to help cure infections of the urinary tract and vaginal yeast as well as to soothe arthritic joints.

If you suffer from an autoimmune disease, echinacea tea may not be right for you because it stimulates the immune system. People who are allergic to plants of the Daisy family may also have trouble tolerating this herb.

Elder

Common Names: Elderberry, pipe tree

The deep purple berries, which make wine, ripen in September yet stay on the tree until late December. However, the flower is the part most often used to make herbal tea. Elder flower produces perspiration in order to bring down a fever, lessen inflammation, and remove toxins. Drink an infusion of both the berries and the flowers when you have a sore throat, cough, or cold. Elder flowers, which taste something like honey, are also drunk in a tea to alleviate the pain of arthritis and symptoms of hay fever. When blended with peppermint, the tea can take away fever blisters.

Be advised that the leaves, roots, and bark of some elder varieties, including the American Elder, which is ubiquitous in North America, contain poisonous alkaloids. Even the unripe berries of this bush can cause cyanide poisoning. The variety to use for tea is the European elder. For this reason, herbalists recommend only using the flowers and ripe berries obtained from an herbal supplier.

Elecampane
Common Names: Elf dock, Helen's flower, horseheal, scabwort, wild sunflower

This tall, hardy perennial is a member of the Aster family. As a couple of its common names suggest, the flowers are bright yellow with white on the inside and they resemble sunflowers. Unlike sunflowers, they emit a delicious violet scent. Also as the common name horseheal reveals, elecampane is used in veterinary medicine.

The fresh leaves can be distilled and made into a wash or facial steam for a fair complexion, but the root is the part used to concoct infusions and decoctions to drink. Elecampane is taken internally primarily to soothe coughs and pulmonary complaints like asthma. It also increases the flow and discharge of bile and produces perspiration in order to bring down a fever, reduce inflammation, remove toxins, increase the body's circulation, and break up obstructions that reduce the body's energy reserves, such as prolonged low-grade fevers or sluggish digestion.

Eyebright
Common Names: Meadow eyebright, red eyebright

This delicate plant of the snapdragon family has two- and three-lobed, tiny white or red flowers. It is semi-parasitic, meaning that it takes nutrition from the roots of neighboring plants. If you want it for your tea garden, plant it in a grassy area away from other botanicals. The parts used for herbal infusions are the flowers, stems, and leaves.

As its name tells, eyebright is one of the best plants to drink as an infusion or to use as an eye wash to cure eye diseases, as it reduces inflammation. By analogy, some believe that a person can drink the tea to produce clarity of vision when endeavoring to enhance concentration. Eyebright is a substance that purifies the blood, removes toxins, and constricts and binds soft tissue to check internal and external secretions like diarrhea and bleeding. The tea can be drunk to soothe a sore throat.

Flax
Common Names: Linseed, lint bells

You may have heard of this blue-flowered plant in connection with uses other than tea making. The fibers have been used to weave linens for ten thousand years, and the oils pressed from the seeds go into making linseed oil, oilcloth, paint, varnish, and linoleum. The seeds also make a very palatable herbal infusion.

Flaxseed is rich in alpha linoleic acid, an essential fatty acid. Since it is a mucilaginous seed, it is considered soothing for coughs and irritated mucus membranes. The soothing nature of flax also makes it effective against constipation and urinary tract infections, but it can also give one flatulence and diarrhea. Flaxseed seems to help shrink the prostate, but some studies have shown that it increases cancer cells of the prostate; so the jury is still out as to the seed's effect on the prostate gland. One thing for certain, flaxseed mimics estrogen in the body, and so can lead to uterine and ovarian cancer if you drink too much of the tea. Never *ever* eat the immature, unripe seeds, as they are highly poisonous.

Ginseng
Common Names: American ginseng, tartar root

This five-leafed perennial herb is found in cool woodlands in North America from Canada and Wisconsin to as far south as Louisiana and Florida. It is a close cousin to Korean or red ginseng, grown mostly in Korea and China, which is reputed to remedy almost every ill that plagues the human body. Since it has been highly sought after for many centuries as a magical panacea and aphrodisiac, the plant is becoming rare. It does not help the situation that ginseng takes six years to mature and a lot of patient hand labor to bring it to market. Ginseng is now on the threatened species list in most states.

Red (Korean) ginseng turns red when processed; American ginseng is white or yellow. A third herb known as Siberian ginseng is a very distant cousin of the other two, but exerts some of the same effects on the human body. It is more easily cultivated, and is therefore cheaper.

The powdered root in an herbal infusion is used principally to counteract age-related disorders such as dementia, senility and rheumatoid arthritis, stress, depression, and minor ailments such as colds and gastrointestinal upsets. In addition to American ginseng, there is a good brand of instant Korean ginseng offered by Prince of Peace. This kind of ginseng is cultivated without herbicides or fertilizers, and so it is considered more or less organic. Open a packet into the bottom of your teacup and add boiling water for instant sizzle. On its own, some herbal tea lovers say that ginseng root tastes bland and parsnip-like. A sweetener with this infusion is recommended.

Hop

Hop is a climbing perennial vine of the hemp family. It is commonly found in wastelands and on roadsides in countries in the northern temperate zone. The flowers are the part used in making tea and beer. Hop flowers are often added to herbal tea recipes along with chamomile to promote a good night's sleep. The flowers calm the nerves and cause both urine and milk to flow. They promote the functioning of the body's systems, maintain health, and increase energy. Hop can be ingested as a preventative when no disease is present. This botanical promotes a healthy appetite and eases indigestion, including gastrointestinal pains. The flowers counteract jaundice and disorders of the bladder, stomach, and liver. Hop is sometimes used in cases of alcoholic delirium tremens as well. The taste is well recognized because the flowers are a flavoring for beer. In an infusion, the flavor is a bit more peppery, and the color is yellow, which makes the hop flower a prime candidate for yellow color healing.

Horehound
Common Names: Hoar-hound, marvel, white horehound

This wooly leafed herb of the Mint family can be found growing in fields and dry wastelands. It has wrinkled, toothed leaves that grow on whitish-gray, woody, square stems and small, whitish flowers in the axils of the leaves. Horehound was a favorite flavoring used by American settlers as an ingredient for candy and cough drops.

Although you can certainly drink it in an infusion, the flavor is bitter and musky. After all, horehound is an ingredient in bitters to stimulate the appetite. If you drink the tea, combine it with a sweeter tasting mint such as spearmint or something spicy like bergamot. Better yet, add something sweet such as licorice or dried cherries, which will add more ingredients for healthy living. The flowers and leaves are the parts used in herbal preparations.

Horehound helps a person cough up mucus, produce a bowel movement, and get a good night's sleep. It has also been ingested to remove intestinal parasites. The herb stimulates the appetite and production of bile. Ancient Greeks administered this herb to treat female infertility, but there is no corroborating scientific evidence to the effect.

Irish Moss
Common Name: Carageen

Irish moss is a type of yellow, green, red, or purple seaweed found on beaches along the North Atlantic coast. In Ireland, it is called "carrageen" after a coastal village where it grows abundantly. During the Irish potato famine, many people saved themselves from starvation by eating it. Besides being an infusion ingredient, the seaweed is used as a filler in some pills and as an emulsifier in facial and body creams.

As with most varieties of seaweed, Irish moss makes an excellent nutritive, promotes the functioning of the body's systems, maintains health, and increases energy. It can be ingested as a preventative when no disease is present because it is rich in many vitamins and minerals such as those found in kelp (see entry). Irish moss also is a remedy for pulmonary, bladder, and kidney disorders.

Jasmine
Common Names: Jessamine, poet's jasmine

The exotically fragrant flowers of this semiperennial, vinelike plant are the part used to prepare herbal tea. More than two hundred species of jasmine exist. The flowers are usually not taken alone; rather they are used to scent green and black teas with their sweetness. The flowers should be consumed fresh, as the dried blossoms carry little fragrance.

Some preliminary studies have been done in Japan and Korea about the vitamin C content of jasmine flowers and their ability to treat hardening of the arteries and promote longevity and a good night's sleep, but more research needs to be done in this area before results can be quoted with confidence.

Juniper
Common Names: Bastard-killer, horse-saver, melmot berries

The berries are the part of this hardwood conifer used to brew infusions. In herbal medicine, juniper is reputed to cure loss of appetite, gastrointestinal and urinary tract infections, geriatric diseases, and to bring on menses. Avoid drinking the herbal infusion if you suffer from kidney disease or are pregnant. Juniper berries taste bitter, but also are spicy and pinelike in a tea. They are often blended with sage for a better taste.

Kelp
Common Name: Sugar wrack

Kelp is a generic name for any of a number of large, brown seaweeds visible only at low tide. They are rich in vitamins A, B, B_2, B_3, B_{12}, C, E, K, aluminum, barium, bismuth, boron, calcium, chlorine, chromium, cobalt, copper, gallium, iodine, magnesium, manganese, molybdenum, phosphorus, sodium, potassium, selenium, sulfur, and zinc.

Kelp makes a wholesome condiment for soups, salads, and meats. You can also add pinches to your herbal teas. This botanical is so valued among herbalists for its vitamin content that it has earned the reputation as a "brain food." It is purported to cleanse arteries and the reproductive system, increase vitality, and remedy eczema, asthma, anemia, headache, and goiter. In an infusion, it tastes bland and somewhat like spinach with a fishlike undertone.

Lady's Mantle

Common Names: Bear's-foot, lion's-foot, nine hooks

The Latin name links this botanical of the Rose family to the ancient art of alchemy and is a tribute to the high repute in which it once was held. Alchemists have attempted to distill essence of lady's mantle to discover the secret of eternal youth without results. The hooked leaves are pleated like a lady's cloak of former times. The plant's clusters of small, yellowish-green flowers bloom from July to August.

All parts of the plant can be used to make an herbal tea, but generally the flowers and leaves are most commonly used. An infusion brewed with lady's mantle and horehound for daily consumption is held by naturopathic healers to increase female fertility. This idea may be based on the alchemical notion that the leaf folds up like an umbrella and retains a drop of morning dew, which was likened to the essence of the womb. What is known for sure is that the infusion helps strengthen muscles, heal internal ruptures, and regularize the shape of the womb after childbirth. This botanical is also used in folk medicine to treat excessive bleeding with periods and diarrhea.

Lady's mantle constricts and binds soft tissue to check internal and external secretions like diarrhea and bleeding. This herb promotes the functioning of the body's systems, maintains health, and increases energy. It can be ingested as a preventative when no disease is present. It also draws water from the kidneys.

Lavender

A shrubby perennial plant of the Mint family, lavender will winter over in cold climates if carefully mulched. The French and Spanish varieties do not produce a superior quality herbal infusion as the English variety.

The name of this plant derives from the word *lavare* in Latin for "to wash." Romans loved washing in lavender oil because of its clean, fresh scent. What they probably did not know is that lavender is an agent that can be applied to the skin to destroy or prevent bacterial growth, sepsis, and putrefaction. If the matter is herbal, it will prevent new growth. For the purposes of this book, you do not need to think about washing in lavender, but rather how it tastes in an infusion and its nutritional value.

The spiky flowers expel mucus from the respiratory tract by promoting coughing. They can also prevent or diminish muscle spasms, cramps, convulsions, and nervous tension. They also help a person get a good night's sleep, so this herb is good to drink in an infusion to calm nerves as well as to relieve heart palpitations. Drink lavender tea to relieve a headache and quiet intestinal gas. Gargle an infusion of the leaves to cure a hoarse throat.

Some naturopaths claim that lavender helps assuage feelings of unresolved guilt, normalize the emotions, and bring heightened awareness. Certainly lavender has a calming, balancing effect on the body. The flowers add a sweetly aromatic, cooling flavor to an herbal tea.

Lemon Balm
Common Names: Melissa, sweet balm, balm

The refreshing, lemony tasting leaves steeped in hot water and cooled with ice make a superior summertime tea. Lemon balm helps reduce fevers and acts as an agent to get a good night's sleep. It also promotes the functioning of the body's systems, maintains health, and increases energy. It can be ingested as a preventative when no disease is present. The infusion is also drunk to lessen nausea, intestinal gas, menstrual cramps, and indigestion. You can also drink the herbal tea to rid yourself of a migraine headache. This herb also regulates menstrual flow and soothes sore throats, aching teeth, and the pain from bee stings.

Lemongrass
You may be familiar with this fine-bladed grass if you enjoy Thai cooking, where it is a staple ingredient. The tall, perennial grass is a native of Africa and Southeast Asia. Lemongrass is added to many medicinal herbal infusions as well as to tea (especially green) to mellow the flavor. The flavor combines well with mint and ginger, and this combination is good for the digestion.

The grass is also drunk in an infusion to bring down fevers, calm nervous tension, and ameliorate arthritic pain. Enthusiasts swear that merely inhaling the steam from the hot tea will cure depression. However, if you are seriously suffering from depression, you should see a medical professional.

Linden
Common Names: Lime tree, tilia

This stately deciduous tree attracts myriad bees in June and July to its ambrosial hanging clusters of yellow blossoms, known as bracts. The bracts and leaves are the parts used in tea making, and the taste is quite pleasant—aromatic, sweet, warm, and apple-like.

Linden is said to have a calming effect on the emotions and is drunk as a digestive to promote the functioning of the body's systems, maintain health, and increase energy. It can be ingested as a preventative when no disease is present. The calming effect linden exudes extends to all the internal organs. Drink the herbal tea to soothe a sore throat and relieve mild kidney and bladder troubles. Linden flowers drunk as a medicinal infusion produce perspiration in order to bring down a fever, lessen inflammation, or remove toxins. Linden is said to help lower blood pressure.

Lovage

Common Names: Italian lovage, garden lovage, sea parsley, scotch lovage

A favorite tall perennial in old English herb gardens, the leaf, root, and fruit are highly aromatic, smelling somewhat like celery. Lovage makes a mild, delicious herbal tea, similar in flavor to angelica.

This aromatic herb brings down fevers, expels gas from the stomach and intestines, causes urine and a woman's period to flow, and stimulates the body's systems. It also contains hefty amounts of vitamin C; so effectively treats deficiency of this vitamin. The medicinal infusion also helps cure colic, flatulence, and bad breath.

Be aware that lovage comprises part of the carrot family and looks similar to deadly water hemlock (also known as poison hemlock and fool's parsley). Do not to attempt to gather it in the wild; buy it at an herb store.

Nettle

Common Name: Stinging nettle

The fresh leaves are incredibly irritating to the skin until they are dried, and this is the part used to make the medicinal herbal infusion. This versatile plant is respected in herbal medicine as an agent that reduces swelling, heat, and pain associated with inflammations. It is a blood purifier, cough promoter, and an agent to constrict and bind soft tissue to check internal and external secretions like diarrhea ad bleeding. Drink the herbal tea to prevent sneezing and itching from seasonal allergies. Nettle also mitigates asthma symptoms, regulates the female reproductive system, and aids weight loss. Because nettle is reasonably rich in iron, this botanical also counteracts anemia and increases mineral assimilation. Nettle contains the flavonoid quercetin, an antioxidant, as well as betasitosterol, which lower absorption of dietary fat, making it a good after-dinner drink.

Nettle tea and extract have been used successfully to treat enlargement of prostate gland (BPH). However, men need to be careful not to drink too much. Nettle contains estrogen, and overindulgence can lead to growth of breasts in men.

If you tire from drinking the herbal tea, pour it on your hair as a rinse to stimulate hair growth. Since fresh nettle is prickly, by analogy, some naturopathic healers claim it helps relieve uncomfortable situations and puts a halt to jealous rumors.

Nutmeg

Although the kernel of this tropical fruit is a well-known culinary spice, it is poisonous in large doses, and may cause miscarriages. If you eat too much nutmeg or drink it brewed in a strong tea, you may feel unable to concentrate, begin to sweat, suffer from heart palpitations, experience pains all over your body, and even suffer from hallucinations. However, these dire consequences only occur with overconsumption. If you use only a few sprinkles in a tea or eggnog as you would do with any spice, you'll be fine. Nutmeg tastes warm, spicy, and sweet. Add a pinch or two to your tea for a nutty, aromatic flavor.

Nutmeg increases the body's circulation and breaks up obstructions that reduce the body's energy reserves, such as prolonged low-grade fevers or sluggish digestion. It is also applied externally to stimulate sore muscles and joints. In small doses, grated nutmeg alleviates symptoms of nausea and heartburn as well. Remember that "small doses" are the operative words here. This spice contains very small amounts of minerals, too, including calcium, copper, iron, magnesium, manganese, potassium, and zinc. The nut also is rich in B complex vitamins, vitamins A and C, folic acid, niacin, and riboflavin.

Oat Straw
Common Name: Groats

Oat straw is the grass on which the oat grain grows. Both grass and grain are used to make the medicinal herbal infusion. Oat straw tea tastes sweet, grassy, and mild. It blends well with chamomile and lavender. If you add a little milk and honey to it, the infusion will fall under the category of white teas in color healing.

The medicinal herbal infusion is drunk to restore strength and vitality after an illness or childbirth, ameliorate nervous exhaustion, and enliven an elderly constitution. Oat straw also prevents or diminishes muscle spasms, cramps, convulsions, and nervous tension. It promotes the functioning of the body's systems, maintains health, and increases energy. It can be ingested as a preventative when no disease is present as a support for the central nervous system. Because it contains silica, it is good for skin, hair, and nails when taken internally.

Passion Flower
Common Names: Apricot vine, maypop, passion vine

As in tea-making, drink a medicinal infusion of all parts of the vine to restore frazzled nerves or gastrointestinal health arising from anxiety. The infusion calms ADHD sufferers and counteracts insomnia. The flowers in an infusion release nervous tension and irritability and nourish the nervous system, and help one get a good night's sleep. Because passion flower prevents or diminishes muscle spasms, cramps, convulsions, and nervous tension, and is a narcotic pain killer, it has been used to alleviate symptoms of Parkinson's disease, nerve pain, and shingles.

Be mindful of the fact that overconsumption of passion flower can trigger drowsiness, nausea, irregular heartbeat, dizziness, and confusion.

Peppermint
Peppermint is one of the many kinds of hardy, leafy perennial mints that grow throughout the temperate zones. This herb thrives in damp, shady patches of the garden. Other common mints used in herbal tea crafting include spearmint, chocolate mint, curly mint, and orange mint, to name a few.

Peppermint essence, extracted by steam distillation, is a good disinfectant and substance that keeps the growth and/or effects of toxic bacteria (one-cell organisms that contain no chlorophyll and some of which can cause disease) in check. This botanical can kill staphylococcus and neutralize the tuberculosis bacillus. A peppermint infusion acts as a decongestant for colds and flu, and alleviates symptoms of morning sickness, dizziness, toothache, headache, vomiting, ulcers, irritable bowel syndrome, bloating, colic, rheumatism, and sore throat.

Raspberry

This prickly bush that grows near water is famous for its sweet red or black berries called hips. The tops before they flower, hips, and leaves are used to prepare an herbal tea that tastes sweetly minty and aromatic. As to raspberry's value in color healing, the leaves turn the liquid in the cup a lovely amber hue. Raspberry leaf is valuable in medicinal infusions. It prevents or diminishes muscle spasms, cramps, convulsions, and nervous tension, and constricts and binds soft tissue to check internal and external secretions like diarrhea and bleeding. It is regarded as one of the best remedies to relieve menstrual cramps, strengthen the uterus, and alleviate nausea during pregnancy. Raspberry promotes the functioning of the body's systems, maintains health, and increases energy. It can be ingested as a preventative when no disease is present. The leaves are also good for stomach upsets, fevers, colds, flu, and canker sores. Moreover, they have been used to treat heart disease. Raspberry hips contain vitamin C. They can sweeten any tea.

Redroot
Common Names: Jersey tea, liberty tea, New Jersey tea, mountainsweet

This three-foot shrub with grayish leaves and white flowers is commonly found from Maine to Florida and Texas. Rather than the root as might be assumed because of its name, the leaves are used to prepare the infusion. It tastes similar to true tea, from the *Camellia sinensis* plant.

Redroot helps relieve diseases of the chest such as asthma, bronchitis, and whooping cough, and it is used as a gargle for throat irritations. It is also drunk to alleviate STD (sexually transmitted disease) conditions such as syphilis and gonorrhea as well as chills, fever, and spasms. The tea or extract taken daily can reduce the size of sebaceous breast cysts or eliminate them entirely.

Rosemary
Common Names: Incensier, old man

The name of this shrubby, tender perennial of the mint family means "sea dew," which refers to the fact that the plant flourishes in poor, dry, calcareous soil near the sea.

This botanical, which tastes crisp and piney in tea, prevents or diminishes muscle spasms, cramps, convulsions, and nervous tension, and constricts and binds soft tissue to check internal and external secretions like diarrhea and bleeding. It produces perspiration in order to bring down a fever, reduce inflammation, or remove toxins. This botanical increases the body's circulation and breaks up obstructions that reduce the body's energy reserves, such sluggish digestion. It is considered a restorative for colds, fevers, and asthma. Rosemary alleviates flatulence and also helps with colic and cleansing of the intestines and kidneys. The medicinal infusion can be taken to lessen muscular pains, especially those arising from sciatica. Try drinking the infusion to cure a headache and recharge your energy. Since rosemary is a nutritive rich in easily assimilated calcium, the herbal tea is a good way to get your daily dose of this mineral without having to swallow a football-size pill.

St. John's Wort

Common Names: Aaron's beard, amber touch-and-heal, rosin rose, goatweed, klamath weed

This favorite botanical of medieval monastery gardens is named for the apostle John because it flowers around June 24, St. John's Day. The woody-stemmed plant with pretty, black-dotted yellow petals is the part used to prepare medicinal and beverage herbal infusions.

Although St. John's wort is drunk as an infusion, it is most often used in extract form. Together with lavender extract and placed in the ear, it is taken as a cure for earache.

The infusion is mainly used to counteract depression and anxiety. It is also a substance that checks the growth and/or effects of toxic bacteria and is an antiviral. St. John's wort constricts and binds soft tissue to check internal and external secretions like diarrhea and bleeding. It can close open wounds, cause urine to flow, soothe nerves, and promote the coughing up of mucus. The extract has been used to treat AIDS/HIV. Because it expels mucus from the respiratory tract by promoting coughing, the herbal tea can be drunk to ease pulmonary congestion and paralysis due to stroke. It is also drunk as a bedwetting preventative.

Use caution when drinking this herbal tea and going outdoors afterwards because St. John's wort increases sensitivity to the sun. This botanical also potentially interacts negatively with a variety of drugs. Check with your doctor before drinking the herbal tea if you are taking any medications for seizure, heart, depression, cancer, HIV, birth control, or anticoagulants.

Skullcap

Common Names: Blue pimpernel, helmetflower, hoodwort, mad-dog weed, scullcap

This creeping botanical with opposite downy leaves receives its generic name from a Latin word meaning "little duck" because the calyx forms a bulging upper lip over the lower lip like a duck's bill. The flower also resembles a type of military helmet with the visor raised; hence another origin of its name.

There are two kinds of skullcap, American and Chinese, and each is used for different reasons. The following addresses American skullcap only.

Herbalists consider this herb of the mint family to be quite valuable; it is prescribed to cure convulsions, neuralgia, and headaches caused by coughing, nervous tension and premenstrual syndrome. A medicinal herbal infusion of the leaf and tops, the parts used, can alleviate symptoms of a hangover. Naturopathic healers claim that this botanical counteracts sterility. Skullcap tea also brings down fevers and is drunk to promote the functioning of the body's systems, maintain health, and increase energy. It can be ingested as a preventative when no disease is present. It contains a significant amount of calcium, magnesium, and potassium. Skullcap tea can help a person get a good night's sleep, decrease inflammation, and guard against hardening of the arteries and stroke. The infusion sometimes is drunk to treat symptoms of epilepsy and other kinds of seizures.

Be aware that large doses of skullcap can cause confusion, dizziness, twitching, and stupor—exactly the symptoms of epileptic seizure it is purported to help cure.

Strawberry

The leaves, which taste cool and strawberry-like in an herbal tea, make a fine tonic for women, and it promotes the functioning of the body's systems, maintains health, and increases energy. The herbal tea can be ingested as a preventative when no disease is present and helps keep a fetus healthy as well. The leaves also constrict and bind soft tissue to check internal and external secretions like diarrhea and bleeding. They help produce a bowel movement, although naturopaths also claim that they stop diarrhea. Modern herbalists prescribe the herbal tea as an appetite promoter and also to stimulate blood cell and hemoglobin formation, although there is no scientific evidence to the effect. Strawberry leaves contain trace amounts of B vitamins, vitamin C, iron, and magnesium. Drink the infusion to boost your immune system.

Valerian

Common Names: All-heal, garden heliotrope, setwell, vandalroot

Valerian is often found in damp spots in woods, hedges, river banks, and at the roadside in the northern temperate zone. The pink or white flowers, standing in clusters atop long stems and flanked by feathery leaves, lend a heavenly scent to the garden. Unfortunately, the part used in healing is the root, which has a peculiar fetid odor.

The herbal tea made from the root prevents or diminishes muscle spasms, cramps, convulsions, and nervous tension. It expels gas from the stomach and intestines, calms nerves, and helps a person get a good night's sleep. It makes an excellent herbal tea for nervous complaints, insomnia, headaches, migraines, hypertension, muscle pains, asthma, chronic fatigue, ADHD, and heart disease. If you only add a small amount, it will impart an interestingly tart flavor to most herbal infusions and teas. Since valerian tends to slow the nervous system, only short-term use is advised.

Vervain

Common Names: Enchanter's plant, fit plant, herb-of-the-cross, Mercury's blood, pigeon's-grass, tears of Isis

This spiky plant displays coarse-toothed or lanced and opposite leaves with five-petal red, purplish or white flowers. The leaves are the part used to prepare medicinal and beverage herbal infusions.

Vervain contains a hefty dose of vitamin K, so it constricts and binds soft tissue to check internal and external secretions like diarrhea and bleeding. The herbal tea also helps expel mucus and causes urine to flow. Drink an infusion to help ease wheezy breathing and cure a headache. Vervain promotes the functioning of the body's systems, maintains health, and increases energy. It can be ingested as a preventative when no disease is present and is a system detoxifier. It also helps in cases of parasites, and worms. Vervain is as useful for depression and nervous disorders as St. John's wort and ginseng, although it is often passed over in favor of those botanicals. Herbalists sometimes prescribe it for cases of gallstones, gout, and jaundice. Because vervain increases blood flow, the infusion can be prescribed to ease the pains of osteoarthritis. In naturopathic healing, this herb is alleged to help overcome feelings of anger and enmity.

Violet
Common Names: Blue violet, English violet

Aromatherapists claim that the blossom's sweet fragrance breaks down the barriers of indifference between people and calms strife. However, the dried leaves are the part used for medicinal infusions. The leaves taken in an herbal tea encourage urine to flow and mucus to be expelled from the chest, and help produce a bowel movement. The herbal tea is prescribed mostly for bronchial conditions.

Be careful not to use the rhizome, as it causes vomiting and diarrhea. Although the rhizome is too strong to drink in a tea, it is alleged, but not scientifically proven, that placing it on the skin will help cure melanomas.

Yarrow
Common Names: Bloodwort, knight's milfoil, sanguinary, stanchgrass

This sunny looking herb with its closely formed yellow, white, or red flower heads and feathery leaves gets some of its common names from the fact that in times gone by, the flowers were used to make an ointment to staunch bleeding and cure wounds. Look for the two- to three-foot tall plant in meadows and on mountainsides.

A medicinal infusion of the leaves and flower tops is drunk to combat bacteria and constrict and bind soft tissue to check internal and external secretions like diarrhea and bleeding. Yarrow induces perspiration in order to bring

down a fever, counteract inflammation, or remove toxins.
The herb expels gas from the stomach and intestines, and
staunches external bleeding. It also helps regulate a woman's menstrual cycle. Yarrow tea is drunk as a remedy for
severe colds and can help alleviate toothache. The taste is
sage-like. Since the brewed liquid looks yellow in the cup,
it can be used in color healing.

Yellow Dock
Common Name: Curled dock

This little plant is often treated as a tenacious garden
weed, but it does possess many virtues in herbal healing.
The term "yellow dock" is a misnomer because the flowers
are reddish brown. The part used is the dried root, which
turns reddish-brown in the teacup, so it can be used either
as a red or brown color in color healing.

Yellow dock is a substance that purifies the blood and
removes toxins, and constricts and binds soft tissue to check
internal and external secretions like diarrhea and bleeding.
It increases the flow and discharge of bile, helps produce
a bowel movement, is a nutritive, promotes the functioning of the body's systems, maintains health, and increases
energy. It can be ingested as a preventative when no disease
is present. Yellow dock is useful in cases of jaundice, iron
deficiency, piles, rheumatism, bleeding from the lungs, and
chronic skin diseases. It is often prescribed by herbalists for
digestive and liver disorders as well as for rheumatism. It
also helps cleanse the lymph glands.

Yerba Santa

Common Names: Bear's weed, consumptive's weed, holy
plant, mountain balm, Palo santo

Yerba Santa grows up to eight feet tall along the roadsides of the West Coast and Baja California. It is easily rec-
ognizable by its pale lavender or blue flowers and leaves that
are covered by a sticky aromatic resin. The leaves are the part
used in medicinal tea preparations. This herb has adapted to
hot, dry conditions, so makes a perfect desert plant.

As to its therapeutic qualities, it is valued as a medicinal herbal infusion to expel phlegm and alleviate bronchial
laryngeal and pulmonary infections, tuberculosis, asthma,
and hay fever. The herbal tea, however, has an initially pungent, spicy flavor, but the aftertaste is soapy sweet. The
leaves are sweet tasting enough that they are used to mask
the taste of more bitter medications.

Plants to Avoid

The following two lists are of botanicals that are poisonous or dangerous for pregnant women, and are not recommended to use in herbal infusions and teas.

Poisonous Botanicals

This list is comprised of plants, which when taken internally, are violent purgatives, cause delirium, hallucinations,
tremors, seizures and diseases like cancer. Some are dangerous to children only, but a few may cause death to anyone.
Do not use them under any circumstances. Some, such as

arnica, are safe to use externally; others such as mugwort or wintergreen can be used in pinches only. Castor bean, for example, will kill you.

- American yew, arnica, beech tree, belladonna, bird's-foot trefoil, bittersweet, black locus, black nightshade, black snakeroot, Bloodroot, Blue Flag, Boldo, Boxwood, Broom, Buckbean, buttercup, butterfly weed, calamus, camphor, Canadian snakeroot, castor bean, celandine, Chinese lantern, Christmas rose, clematis, coltsfoot, comfrey, common groundsel, cottonseed, daffodil, datura, death camas, deers' tongue, desert plume, English holly berries, ergot, figwort, forget-me-not, foxglove, fumitory, goldenseal, hedge mustard, hellebore, hemp dogbane, henbane, herb mercury, horse chestnut, Indian pink, Indian tobacco, iris, jaborandí tree, lady's-slipper, larkspur, lesser periwinkle, lily of the valley, lobelia, mahuang, marsh marigold, mayapple, milkweed, mistletoe, monkshood, moonseed, mountain ash berries, mountain laurel, mugwort, nightshade, opium, poppy, pennyroyal, peyote, periwinkle, pokeweed, prickly poppy, quassia, red baneberry, rosebay rhododendron, soapwort, sorrel, southernwood, spindletree, squaw root, strychnine tree, sweet coltsfoot, sweet flag, sweet woodruff, tansy, thuja, Virginia snakeroot, wallflower, water hemlock,

white false hellebore, white mustard, white
snakeroot, wild cherry, wild licorice, winter cress,
wintergreen, wormseed, wormwood, yellow flag,
yellow jessamine, yellowroot

Botanicals Harmful to Ingest During Pregnancy

Every woman's physical constitution is different, so what
one pregnant woman may tolerate well, another will not
abide. Most of the botanicals on this list are safe to consume for those who are not pregnant. Almost all of the following botanicals are listed on medical websites as being
potentially harmful to mother and fetus. In many cases,
not enough research has been done; doctors need to be
very careful about pregnancy and nutrition. Here are listed
only common potentially harmful tea making botanicals.
Throughout this manual, others have been mentioned.
Obviously, you should not consume any of the botanicals
on the previous page's "poisonous" list either. For a complete list, check out pregnancy websites such as www.
motherlove.com and www.naturalark.com.

The following botanicals make the list because they
affect the hormones, are too strong or irritating, or bring
on bleeding or contractions:

- Aloe vera, angelica, barberry, bee balm, black cohosh, blue cohosh, black walnut, blessed thistle, borage, buckthorn, cascara sagrada, catnip, chaste tree berry, chicory, damiana, dong quai, elecampane, fenugreek, feverfew, gentian, goldenseal, horehound, juniper berries, licorice, lovage, motherwort, Oregon grape root, osha, parsley, pennyroyal, rosemary, sage, sarsaparilla, Siberian ginseng, thyme, tumeric, yarrow

Six

Ailments from A to Z and Teas to Help

This chapter lists common ailments and some suggested teas and herbal teas to help prevent and support them when they do occur. The key words here are "prevent and support." These suggestions are not meant to be cures; they are suggested because they can help mitigate symptoms. The list is not exhaustive, by all means, but it does provide a reasonable number of choices. Look for more extensive information about these teas where they are described in other chapters of this book.

Alertness—Assam black tea, Constant Comment black tea, English breakfast black tea, Irish breakfast black tea, chocolate tea, green tea

Allergies—dong quai, nettle, plantain, honeybush, rooibos

Anti-aging—white tea, rooibos, ginseng, oat straw

Anxiety—passionflower, St. John's wort, valerian, hawthorn berries

Appetite suppressant—black tea, green tea, white tea, cinnamon, fennel, hibiscus, chai tea, parsley, kelp

Arthritis—rosehips, orange peel, alfalfa, bergamot, blessed thistle, elder flowers, vervain, burdock root, devil's claw root, flaxseed, licorice, nettle, turmeric

Asthma—nettle, plantain, alfalfa, anise, elecampane, rosemary, yerba santa, red clover

Autoimmune diseases—gingko

Backache—devil's claw, cinnamon, clary sage

Bad breath—clove, anise, fennel, lovage, peppermint, spearmint

Bedwetting—ginseng, chamomile, St. John's wort

Bladder infection—angelica, buchu, corn silk, couch grass, cranberry, dandelion root and leaf, hop, Houjicha green tea, Irish moss, juniper berries, linden bracts, nettle, parsley, vervain, white tea

Blood circulation and pressure (to lower it)—alfalfa, ginger, angelica, cinnamon, hibiscus, red clover, black tea, chocolate tea, puerh tea, althea root, lemon, rosehips

Bone problems (including osteoporosis)—black tea, cat's claw, Matcha green tea, honeybush, rosehips

Breast cancer and precancerous lesions—redroot, green tea (more scientific studies need to be done)

Bronchitis—Echinacea, redroot

Cellulite—green tea (all kinds), yellow tea

Cerebral problems (Alzheimer's dementia, Parkinson's, brain tumor, etc.)—black tea, green tea, gingko, ginseng, passionflower, licorice

Cholesterol (High LDL)—black tea, twig green tea, white tea, basil, ginger, honeybush, blackberry leaf

Cold—angelica, catnip, Sunshine Dragon green tea, echinacea, elder flowers, ginger, ginseng, guaraná, hibiscus, lemon balm, lemon peel, licorice root, orange peel, peppermint, raspberry leaf, redroot, rosehips, spearmint, thyme, yarrow

Constipation—althea root, burdock root, chicory, ginger root, fennel, horehound, lemon peel, licorice root, raspberry leaves, strawberry leaves, violet leaves, yellow dock; senna leaf tea can be used sparingly, but be aware that it has a strong laxative effect

Depression—ginseng, bergamot, gingko, St. John's wort, orange peel, lemon peel, lemongrass

Diabetes—black tea, bilberry, burdock, green tea, juniper, rooibos

Diarrhea—agrimony, bilberry, blackberry leaf, blueberry leaf, caraway, chai tea, chamomile, cinnamon, lemon verbena, licorice root, peppermint, raspberry leaf, rose petals, spearmint

Digestion (indigestion; heartburn; stomach, colon, and intestinal trouble)—angelica, bergamot, cat's claw, chamomile, Darjeeling black tea, fennel, ginger, ginseng, bancha green tea, hop, Keemun black tea, orange pekoe black tea, passionflower, peppermint, puerh tea, rooibos, sage, spearmint

Eczema—blessed thistle, chamomile, gingko, burdock, kelp, calendula, yellow dock

Esophageal cancer—green tea (any kind, but Dragonwell is suggested as a good choice)

Exhaustion/Fatigue/Overwork—dandelion root, gingko, ginseng, guaraná, kelp, licorice, oat straw, passionflower, peppermint, rosemary, sage, valerian

Fever—catnip, borage, elderflower, feverfew, lovage, yarrow

Flatulence—Chai tea, cinnamon, angelica, sage, rosemary, lovage, cinnamon, rosemary, thyme, borage

Flu and other common viruses—Earl Grey black
tea, Pi Lo Chun green tea, Pouchong green tea,
thyme, honeybush, white tea, St. John's wort, hops,
echinacea, ginseng, raspberry hips, hibiscus

Fluid retention—bergamot, black, green, or white tea
(any kind), dandelion root, hibiscus, lady's mantle

Focus (lack of)—Assam black tea, English breakfast
black tea, Irish breakfast black tea, gingko, rooibos
and honeybush (taken together)

Gout—devil's claw, vervain

Hair loss—Matcha green tea, alfalfa, horsetail, nettle,
oat straw

Hay fever—alfalfa, yerba santa, elder flowers

Headache—black tea, green tea, basil, chocolate tea,
cinnamon, feverfew, ginger, gingko, kelp, lavender,
lemon balm, lemongrass, peppermint, rosemary,
spearmint, vervain

**Heart trouble (heart attack, stroke, hardening of
arteries, etc.)**—Ceylon black tea, hibiscus, kelp,
gingko, hawthorn, rooibos, calendula, skullcap

Hemorrhage—alfalfa, blackberry, goldenseal, lady's
mantle, nettles, shepherd's purse, yarrow

Insomnia—anise, catnip, chamomile, hops, orange
peel, passionflower, St. John's wort, valerian

Joint aches and inflammation—basil, bergamot, cardamom, celery seed, echinacea, ginger, lemon verbena, licorice, nettle, parsley, rooibos, rosehips and petals, turmeric

Kidney trouble—black tea, dandelion root, Irish moss, linden, chai tea, rosemary, basil, ginger

Liver trouble—burdock root, calendula, chicory, dandelion root, elder flowers, hop, kelp, milk thistle, nettles, rosehips, rosemary, sencha green tea, thyme, yellow dock

Lung trouble (including infections, chest pains due to bronchial infections)—anise, elecampane, honeybush, red clover, ginger root, lemon ginger green tea, horehound, Irish moss, thyme, yellow dock, althea root (marshmallow), orange peel, vervain, nettle, yerba santa

Memory—English breakfast black tea, Irish breakfast black tea, lapsang souchong black tea, Constant Comment black tea, ginseng, gingko, licorice, lemon verbena, cinnamon

Menstruation—nettle, juniper, bergamot, blessed thistle, raspberry hips, parsley, sage, alfalfa, black cohosh, peppermint, calendula

Migraine—valerian, feverfew, lemon balm, thyme

Motion sickness, nausea—angelica, anise, chamomile, ginger, lavender, lemon balm, lemon verbena, peppermint, raspberry hips, spearmint

Nervousness—valerian, vervain, red clover, passionflower, hawthorn berries, catnip, thyme

Pancreatic disease—green tea

Prostate trouble—black tea, white monkey's paw green tea, nettle, saw palmetto berries, damiana, flaxseed (more scientific research needs to be done on this last suggestion)

Psoriasis—blessed thistle, yellow dock, calendula, lavender

Rheumatism—orange peel, ginseng, devil's claw, peppermint, yellow dock

Sciatica—devil's claw, rosemary

Skin aging—white tea, gingko, calendula, chamomile, dandelion leaf, hibiscus, honeybush, oat straw, rooibos, rosehips

Skin cancer—rooibos and honeybush (taken together), violet leaves

Sore throat—althea root, borage, honeysuckle flowers, lavender, sage, slippery elm

Stress—catnip, ginseng, hops, lavender, lemon verbena, licorice, linden, passionflower, oat straw, black tea (any kind), green tea (any kind), white tea (any kind), rosehips and petals, skullcap, valerian

Toothache, decay, and gum disease (gum disease can also indicate cardiovascular problems)—matcha green tea, calendula, cinnamon, clove, lavender, lemon balm, peppermint, spearmint, yarrow, blackberry leaf, spearmint, calendula

Vision problems—gingko, calendula, eyebright, clary sage, bilberry

Weight gain—kelp

Weight loss, fat metabolism—black tea (any kind), gunpowder green or young hyson green tea, white tea (any kind), puerh tea, alfalfa, cinnamon, fennel, guaraná, honeybush, nettle, oolong tea (any kind), red clover, chai tea, kelp, vanilla (inhaled)

Women's disorders (including ovaries, uterus, premenstrual syndrome, menopause, pregnancy, cancer)—black tea, green tea, yellow tea, white tea (any kind of those teas if they can be tolerated in pregnancy), honeybush, raspberry hips, nettles, kelp, clary sage, red clover, dong quai, nettle, black cohosh (menopause only)

Seven

How to Brew Tea

This chapter discusses how to brew medicinal and beverage teas and herbal teas. Items needed to brew both single cups and pots of tea are covered as well as additives such as sugar, lemon, and milk. Storage tips are offered. The chapter ends with a discussion of how to brew herbal infusions and decoctions.

Items Required

You do not have to lay out a substantial monetary investment to become a skilled tea steeper. You have already learned the hard part, which is choosing the appropriate teas. Now all you need is water, a pot for heating it, a teapot for steeping the brew, a cup, a saucer, a spoon, a napkin to catch spills, and an infuser. And of course you will need a heat source—that goes without saying. Here are the basics.

Water

Cold, filtered tap water makes the best cup of tea. Experts agree that bottled water, because it is less oxygenated, can cause a brew to taste flat. The oxygen contained in filtered tap water makes the tea taste sweeter and more flavorful, especially if you are brewing a white, yellow, or green variety.

There is also a controversy surrounding bottled water. You may have heard how landfills are overflowing with nonrecyclable plastic bottles. Thousand of tons of these containers end up in the oceans every year, polluting the water and endangering marine life. Worse, many of these bottles are made from polyethylene terephthalate, PETE or PET for short, as the bottles containing these substances are required to be labeled. PETE relates to bisphenol A, phtalates, and antimony (a component of flame retardants and batteries). What do these big words mean to the bottled water drinker?

Over time, the chemicals in the packaging can leach into the liquids contained in the bottles, especially acidic liquids such as orange juice and tea. The chemicals can disturb the body's endocrine system, disrupt hormones like testosterone and estrogen, and cause fertility problems. They can increase levels of blood cholesterol and contribute to neurological, behavioral, and immune system disorders. Health-aware bottling companies have switched to safe plastic or gone back to glass, but such manufacturers are few and far between.

Bottled water usually comes from municipal systems anyway. So consumers pay many times more for something they could have gotten free from the tap. Worse, when bottled water has been tested, some of it has been found to contain carcinogens, bacteria, and chemicals. For all these reasons, properly filtered, cold (not hot from the tap), oxygenated tap water seems to be the most wholesome, flavorful, and cheapest choice.

Vessel

Next you will need a heat-proof vessel in which to heat the water. The top choice is an old-fashioned teakettle. A wide-mouthed pot will do in a pinch, but you will probably end up spilling a lot of water. The only kinds of pots not recommended are those made from aluminum or with Teflon coating on the inside. Both can leach into the water and affect the taste and your health. Do not reboil old water left over in the pot as it makes the tea taste lifeless and a bit tinny. And remember to keep your vessel in good repair.

Cup

Any kind of cup will do except those made from plastic. Some tea drinkers also dislike Styrofoam. However, tea tastes equally delectable sipped from a porcelain cup or quaffed from a mug.

The small glazed bowls used in Asia are perfect for enjoying multiple steepings of tea. Some drinkers prefer glass mugs because they like to watch what tea masters call "the agony of the leaves"; that is, the process whereby the leaves unfurl and move around in the cup, ever changing color until just the right hue is achieved. The appropriate hue, as you have learned, is important for color healing.

Saucer

One addition you might consider, even if you are drinking from a mug and not from a teacup, is a saucer. Place it on top of the cup or mug to condense the tea's essential oils back into the cup. This is especially important when you brew herbal botanicals other than *Camellia sinensis* for medicinal purposes. Saucers are practical, too, in that they catch spills. For the same reason, you may want to keep a napkin within reach and a spoon as well, especially if you add sweetener, lemon, or milk.

Teapot

A short answer to the best kind of pot for steeping is to use whatever is available. Even dunking a teabag in a mug makes a fast way of preparation. It might taste like an astringent stew and certainly lacks panache, but sometimes the quickest way suffices. Besides, as Edward Bramah, world-renowned tea expert and founder of the Bramah Tea and Coffee Museum in London, once said, today's average teabag is designed to infuse in less than fifty seconds, so teabags make good choices for people on the go.

Of course the finest receptacle for steeping tea is a proper teapot. Some beautiful teapots of all shapes and sizes are available. Some are square, others round, oblong, large, small, multi-colored, embossed, plain, thematic, made from porcelain, clay, wood, glass, and other materials. Each individual pot enhances the tea's flavor in a different way and adds to the wonder and delight of taking tea. As with teacups, avoid plastic and aluminum both for the strange taste they impart to the tea and for the carcinogens that may leak into the brew.

When shopping for a basic teapot, here are some points to consider. First and foremost, pick up the pot. While the store clerk probably will not let you brew tea in it, you can mimic pouring. Judge how the pot feels in your hand. Is the handle big enough to fit several fingers comfortably around it? Does the lid fit snugly over the opening so you will not need to hold it in place while you pour?

As to the opening, is it wide enough to hold an infusion basket and to insert a brush or sponge to clean inside? A high spout is a plus because it enables you to fill the pot to the top. Now check the base. A wide base will keep a pot stable no matter where you set it.

Glass teapots are interesting. As with glass mugs, they allow you to monitor the tea's strength and watch the mesmerizing color intensify as the leaves steep. You will know right away when the tea is steeped just the way you like it by observing the pot.

Yixing teapots, fabricated from special Zisha clay, are deemed by many tea masters to be the most perfect tea brewing vessels in the world. They come from the Yixing region of China northwest of Shanghai and are cherished by collectors for their simplicity and beauty. You may recognize Yixing pots as the ones traditionally used in to prepare tea the Chinese Gung Fu way. Their reputation is due to the fact that these pots retain heat well and do not expand during firing. If you purchase Yixing, you will need a separate pot for each type of tea, as the porous clay cures after repeated use, and seasons each successive pot of tea with accumulated flavor.

Although Yixing pots are simply styled, they are available in a variety of shapes and sizes, including round and square. Often they sport animal designs, the most popular being a dragon. You can find a turtle, phoenix, or tall dragon among other critter varieties. Most Asian or Eastern teapots are small, holding only up to ten ounces of water.

Another Chinese invention, the gaiwan, has remained popular since the sixteenth century. This versatile tool can be used as a teapot, tea taster's cup, teacup, or even as a saucer. The porcelain comes in various sizes, with the smallest holding a mere three to five ounces.

Colorful tetsubin Japanese teapots are cast iron pots ideal for brewing green teas. They retain more heat longer than any other kind of teapot. Because the inside is enameled, they are easy to clean. Since the Tetsubin are Asian- or Eastern-style pots, sizes are fairly small. A typical pot holds eleven ounces, but a sixteen-ounce size is also available (if not a bit heavy). Colors include red, green, blue, and black, and each comes with a stainless steel infuser.

For a more English-style teapot, you might like a Chatsford. This glazed earthenware pot stands somewhat taller than a Japanese pot, and comes in white, brown, blue, green, and yellow. You can purchase a small pot that holds two cups or a larger four-cup version. Chatsfords usually are provided with a removable mesh infuser.

Of all English-style teapots, undoubtedly the most beloved is the legendary Brown Betty. Its rise to fame came about because of three simultaneous and related occurrences along with a fourth, ineffable factor. Back in the mid-eighteenth century, the earls of Fitzwilliam, the Rockinghams, who were giants of industry, rolled out a new line of earthenware pottery. This pottery was characterized by a distinctive glossy brown glaze, whose chemical formula consisted, in part, of manganese and iron.

At the same time, a new type of teapot, round and stout and made from red clay, was being manufactured in Stoke-on-Trent, the pottery capital of England. The stylish shape, coupled with the Rockingham brown glaze, came along at the time when tea-drinking was spreading throughout Britain and Ireland. The Brown Betty, as this teapot was called, became fashionable. It got an even more regal nod later from Queen Victoria, who declared that this type of pot made the very "best cup of tea." This last phrase encompasses the fourth factor that characterizes the Brown Betty. To this day, many British swear that the Brown Betty, indeed, produces the very finest and healthiest cup of tea. Certainly the trace amounts of manganese and iron that come from the pot's material provide additional minerals to the tea. Good source for purchasing teapots include: www.teavana.com/tea-products/teapots-teapot-sets and www.republicoftea.com/teapots/c/52/.

Infuser

You will need an infuser or strainer to hold the loose leaves so they do not escape into the cup. The best infusers are made from metal mesh or are bamboo baskets. Other choices include tea balls, fabric tea socks, and paper filters. Never pack leaves tightly into the infuser. You want to leave room for them to unfurl and move freely through the water. One infuser to avoid is the kind designed for a single cup of tea shaped like two half-teaspoons and wired so that they open and close. This type of infuser does not allow enough room for the leaves to unwind and so produces an inferior-tasting cup of tea.

Tea Cozy

A tea cozy (also spelled "cosy") makes a nice but unnecessary addition. It is like a small quilted jacket that keeps a teapot and the tea inside warm.

How to Prepare a Beverage Infusion

Most experts agree that the best way to enjoy a fine cup of tea is to prepare an infusion. Although a beverage infusion differs from a medicinal infusion in that it is often brewed for less time, you can still derive benefits for healthy living from a beverage in fusion. In short, preparing a beverage infusion consists of boiling one cupful of water, pouring it over one teaspoonful of fresh leaves, and steeping the brew for up to five minutes. If you steep it in a pot, add an extra teaspoonful "for the pot" and pour into teacups. Add sweetener and milk or lemon, if desired. Stir once, and drink immediately. The foregoing is the short answer to brewing a beverage infusion, and if you are satisfied with it, move on to the section on sweeteners. For those who wish more precise instructions, continue reading.

Two basic methods for steeping tea depend on whether you take your tea Asian or Eastern or Western style. In Asia, the teapot and cups are small, but many more leaves are used. This is because the steeping time is quite short—generally thirty seconds to one minute, and the leaves are meant to be resteeped up to eight times.

How to Prepare a Single Cup of Tea

In contemporary Western societies, most people do not have time to prepare a big pot of tea to enjoy at their leisure. They prefer to take their tea by the single cupful or, more likely, by the mug. Following are some suggestions for how to prepare a first-rate single cup of tea.

Some tea masters recommend that you never bring the water to a full boil. They tell you to heat the water until it begins to form bubbles, and if it comes to a boil by mistake, let the water cool for one minute before pouring it over the leaves. Otherwise you risk scorching the leaves and ending up with a dull-tasting brew. Others instruct to bring the pot to a gentle boil, especially for the stronger blacks and puerhs. Following this section is a table of recommended water temperatures and steeping times for all kinds of teas. You will find a range of temperatures and brewing times. In the end, it all boils down (ha) to individual taste.

Besides arguing over temperatures and brewing times, some tea masters cannot even seem to agree on how to pour the water. Most advocate pouring it directly over the leaves. They warn against sprinkling leaves into a cup already full of hot water because the leaves will tend to float on top and not infuse properly. A few renegades give the opposite recommendation and insist that you should place the leaves or teabag into the hot water after it is poured.

Figuring out how long to steep your cup of tea can be equally confusing. A sure way to demystify this conundrum is to read the directions on the side of the package. If none exist, ask a knowledgeable salesperson where you bought the tea. If you still cannot find an answer, consult the following chart that has been culled from various sources.

For each cup of tea or beverage herbal tea, use half a teaspoon of dried leaves or one level teaspoon of fresh leaves. If the tea leaves are quite large, as in some whole leaf teas, you might want to use a heaping teaspoonful. Splash hot water into the cup or mug and drain it to warm the cup before pouring your tea. This procedure holds true for a teapot as well.

....

Recommended Water Temperatures and Steeping Times

Kind of Tea	Amount of Tea per Cup	Water Temperature	Steeping Time
White	1 tsp.	175-180 or 185 F (80-85 C)	1-2 min. or 7–9 min.
Yellow	1 tsp.	195 F (90 C)	1-2 or 3 min.
Green	1 tsp.	150-160 or 175 F (65-80 C)	1-2 min. 2 ½-3 min. or 3-4 min.
Oolong	½ tsp.	190 or 195 F (86-90 C)	2-4 min. or 3 min. exactly. or 3-6 min.
Black	½ tsp.	205 or 212 F (96 or 100 C)	3-5 min.
Puerh	½ tsp.	205 F (96 C)	3-4 min. or 5-8 min.

....

Some people complain about green tea having a bitter taste. People may get this idea because they brew it incorrectly. Green tea can be something of a prima donna, no doubt, but when it is brewed correctly, it is considered to taste grassy, slightly sweet, pliable on the tongue, delicious, and healthy. Experiment by first covering the cup, and then brewing for half of the recommended time. Taste the tea and steep a little longer until you get the flavor you like best.

Brewing Iced Tea

To make iced tea, prepare a double strength infusion according to the table on the previous page. Double-strength is recommended because the tea will be diluted by the ice. Strain away the leaves and cool the tea to room temperature. Pour over ice cubes in glasses, and serve. Sprigs of mint, lavender, lemon balm or a lemon slice make refreshing garnishes. The ice cubes should be made from pure, filtered tap water like the tea.

Teabag Tea

Most tea histories will tell you that the teabag was invented in 1908 by tea merchant William Sullivan. To sell more tea, he packaged samples in small silk bags. Matrons of the city's bourgeoisie were so enchanted by the little bags that they clamored to have all of their tea orders filled in that way. Today some gourmet tea companies like Mighty Leaf still offer teabags in little silk sacks.

Nobody really knows who first dunked a bag of botanicals into hot water and drank the end result, but many claim the honor. For example, in another legend, the Chippewa are said to have invented the teabag by placing herbs on very thin strips of bark and tying them up before immersing the bark bags in the boiling water.

In Britain, teabags rose to popularity after World War II. Before the war, the British infused loose, rolled-leaf tea. After the war, coffee producers introduced soluble coffee powder to the market so consumers could make coffee instantly. The tea trade responded to this coffee challenge by using CTC (cut, tear, and curl) machines instead of rollers to produce a granulated tea that would infuse as quickly as coffee. No matter what tea purists may feel, today most of the tea sold in Britain (and in the US, for that matter), is the bagged variety.

The very smallest leaves and tiniest broken bits left over from the manufacturing process are called fannings and dust. Though the term "dust" may sound unappetizing, you can rest assured that the manufacturers do not scoop dust from the factory floor and spoon it into teabags. Many of these small leaves can be quite palatable. In fact, this is probably the kind of tea with which you are most familiar because fannings and dust are usually reserved for teabags. Some tea drinkers prefer bagged tea because it infuses rapidly with no fuss and has a bracing flavor. However, because teabag tea uses CTC leaves, some health benefits are lost.

To steep bagged tea, pour hot water over the bag and let it steep for two to five minutes only, depending on the kind of tea you are drinking and the strength you desire. For white tea, two minutes is suggested, for green tea, three minutes, and for black tea, four to five. Steeping times are very much up to individual taste, so it is suggested you experiment and choose the steeping times you like best. Remove the bag—never squeeze it to wring out the last of the acerbic-tasting tea—and add lemon or sweetener or milk. Stir once, and your tea is ready to drink.

As tea rises to prominence in the beverage industry, it comes as no surprise that resourceful entrepreneurs are inventing ingenious teabag sidelines. One such businessman is Barry Cooper, founder of Cooper's Tea Company. His latest invention is a tea pod that will fit inside a Melitta One:One coffee filtering machine. Pop one of his tea pods into the top of a One:One machine and a 12- or 16-ounce glass of hot tea shoots out the bottom in around half a minute. Cooper sells his pods to a company that supplies Bed Bath & Beyond, JC Penney, Sears, and Target. If you do not have a Melitta One:One machine you can also get tea in Keurig K-cups. They can be used in Keurigs or other machines that use K-cups. There are K-cups that you can fill with your own coffee, and presumably with your own loose leaf tea.

Bagging Your Own

There are some good reasons to occasionally bag your own tea. In the first place, when you do, you will know that the tea is as fresh as possible, and freshness equates to healthy living. Also when you make your own tea, especially your own herbal blends stored in containers, the heavier ingredients will invariably accumulate in the bottom of the jar. Filling a bag will ensure that all of the ingredients make it into the packet. Pop the filled bags back into the containers where the blend came from and they will stay fresh and ready to use.

You can buy empty teabags for pennies at most tea emporiums and online. Place one teaspoonful of your personal recipe (no more, for you want to give the leaves room to unfurl) into the little porous paper sack and seal it shut with a hot iron. You do not even need to use an iron if you do not mind the tea occasionally leaking out. Just fold over the bag, and your personal teabag is ready for action.

Storing Tea

Tea leaves are a delicate commodity. This distinction gives them the elusive, subtle aroma and flavor so loved by tea enthusiasts. It also means that tea leaves readily absorb aromas from whatever happens to be hanging around their vicinity, good or bad. To avoid contaminating your tea leaves, do not store tea near your spice rack, and if possible keep them away from light, heat, and moisture. It goes without saying that you should never freeze or refrigerate the fragile leaves because tea does not tolerate temperature extremes. On the other hand, some fresh herbs freeze well. Basil is an example; dill, another, and most seeds can be frozen, too.

No matter what kind of tea or herb you purchase and whether you buy it bagged or loose, always store your tea in an airtight container to preserve freshness. Ceramic or classic tea tins work well. A traditional way to store tea is in a small wooden tea chest. In centuries gone by, tea was a rare and precious commodity. The lady of the house always locked up her tea in one of these chests so as not to tempt servants. If you are lucky enough to find one of these old chests at an antiques fair, perhaps the wood will still retain some of the aroma of tea leaves past and impart its light scent of yesteryear to your treasured tea leaves.

If you store tea properly, it will last for a fairly long time. Some tea masters recommend keeping white, yellow, and green teas for no longer than three to six months, oolongs for six to nine months, and black teas for no more than one year before you toss it. If your tea goes stale sooner and you wish to revive it, spread a thin layer of it on a sheet of paper for a few hours in a well-aired room.

Sweeteners

Sugar

As you read in chapter 1 about sweet tea and bubble tea, many tea drinkers like to add sweetener to every type of tea. Sugar is usually the favorite. Most table sugar comes from sugar cane or sugar beets. Cane sugar probably originated in South and East Asia, where it has been cultivated since at least 1000 BCE. Europeans came late to the game and did not start using it until after the Middle Ages. Until then, their major sweetener was honey. For them and others, sources of sweetness were found in malt, milk, sorghum grass, maple, palm trees, grapes, and other fruit.

Types of sugar you are likely to find on your supermarket shelves include:

- **Granulated (white)**—This highly refined cane or beet sugar is the most commonly used table sugar.

- **Superfine (also called "caster sugar")**—It is extra-granulated and dissolves easily in iced drinks.

- **Confectioner's (also called powdered or icing sugar)**—Sugar is granulated and then crushed and mixed with cornstarch. It is often used in frosting but does not dissolve well in tea.

- **Brown**—Both the light and dark colors are made from highly refined sugar that has been sprayed with molasses. It is mostly used in baking rather than in beverages.

- **Demerara**—In some quarters, the large, golden crystals that dissolve readily in tea and coffee are considered gourmet quality. White sugar crystals, also known as "decorating sugar," are four times the size of granulated crystals, and are used for ornamentation on cakes and other desserts.

- **Turbinado**—If you are lucky, you may find turbinado at your grocery store. It consists of raw, partially processed cane sugar, where the molasses is only partly washed off. Therefore, it actually contains many of the nutrients of molasses, including vitamin B_6, potassium, magnesium, and manganese. Turbinado's slightly nutty, spicy flavor tastes heavenly in tea and other beverages.

- **Muscovado**—This very dark brown and coarse substance is even less processed than turbinado and has a strong molasses flavor. It is a challenge to flush out muscovado in this country, but it is widely available in Latin America. Look for it in the US at Latino food markets. Muscovado also contains the nutrients listed under "Turbinado" that are not in other sugars.

Sugar makes much of what people eat and drink taste better and certainly provides energy in the form of carbohydrates. But as is the case of salt, it turns out to be too much of a good thing. The average American consumes 21 to 22 teaspoonfuls of sugar daily, adding 320 to 350 calories to our diets. No wonder Americans are packing on the pounds! You might not think you eat very much sugar, but it sneaks into much of your food as an additive you might not even taste.

Besides contributing to obesity, sugar can cause all kinds of health problems such as hyperactivity in children, allergies, eczema, low human growth hormone levels (a factor in premature aging), osteoporosis, diabetes, lessened protein absorption, high LDL (bad) cholesterol, vaginal yeast infections, and lowered resistance to bacterial infections.

Even though there is a downside to sugar, there is an upside, too. Besides giving you energy, sugar is a good substance to eat to bulk up if you are on the undernourished side. You can also enjoy tea-infused sugars that will provide some of the nutrition found in regular tea. Tea sugars make tasty treats, summer or winter, and can be added to tea hot or cold. Or you can use them to impart a tea-like flavor to other drinks, dessert dishes, and marinades.

You can infuse sugar with any kind of dried tea leaf. Black tea works best because it has the spiciest flavor, and the taste you get with an infused sugar will always be mild, at best. You can also create infusions using herbal tea botanicals. Popular flavors include jasmine flowers, rose petals and buds, lavender, rosemary, anise, lemon balm, cinnamon, and a variety of citrus peels such as orange, lemon, tangerine, and lime. One appropriate tea to infuse into sugar is Constant Comment because of the tangy aroma of the spicy peels.

Making tea-infused sugars is easy. Use demerara sugar because the crystals are large, the sugar is less processed, and the taste is good. Granulated organic sugar is also a good choice. You can infuse any kind of sugar except the powdered variety, which is quite messy.

Pour one cup of sugar into an airtight container, such as a tin or Mason jar. Take a small muslin bag and fill it with at least two tablespoons of dried tea and/or dried herbs, flowers, seeds, or peels. The purpose of the muslin bag is to prevent bits of organic material from leaking into the sugar.

Put the filled bag into the sugar and use a mortar and pestle to release the essences. Cover with some of the sugar, and grind some more. Now close the container and wait. Stir the sugar and sample it every day until you obtain the flavor and strength you desire—usually around one week. When the sugar tastes just right to you, remove the teabag and fertilize your azaleas and camellias with the spent leaves.

Honey

Some people prefer to add honey to their tea. This natural product of bees has been a favored sweetener, probably since the first human worked up the courage to stick a hand into a hive. The viscous and ethereally fragrant substance can be yellow, white, brown, orange, green, purple—even black—thick or thin, strong or mild, depending on which flowers the bees have visited. If you have a chance to visit a gourmet store, try honey made from orange blossoms, raspberries, sage, eucalyptus, rosemary, or heather. Be aware that some honeys can be poisonous or narcotic, depending on the flowers from which the nectar is gathered. Oleander honey, for example, falls under the deadly poisonous category. Also a lot of honey these days comes from China, where foodstuffs are not always monitored as carefully as in the US.

In the health department, honey is better for you than sugar, but only marginally. It contains approximately the same amount of fructose and glucose, so it is not a good choice for diabetics. Also some vegans tend to reject honey because they abhor the mistreatment of bees. The calories are more or less the same, too, so honey will not help you lose weight. The best that can be said for it is that it is a less processed product. Honey also has some antioxidant properties that fight bacteria, and you can drink it in tea with lemon to suppress a cough or ease a sore throat.

Clover honey is one of the most readily available and better-tasting choices for tea. It does not quite substitute for sugar, though, because of its consistency, but it is worth taking time to experiment.

Agave Nectar

Here is another sweetener that some health gurus tout as a healthy alternative to sugar. Agave sap is extracted from the core of the Blue Agave, a spiky Mexican succulent that looks something like an aloe vera or yucca plant. The core, which is called a "pineapple," is huge, weighing between fifty and a hundred pounds. After harvesting, it is then filtered and heated to produce the nectar, or syrup. Because low temperatures (under 118 degrees) are used to extract the nectar, many natural food fans consider agave a raw food. Those same vegans who do not wish to harm bees by disturbing their nests accept agave as a number one alternative to honey. They also point to the fact that agave ranks fairly low on the glycemic index, meaning that it does not readily raise blood sugar levels.

What agave enthusiasts do not mention is that the reason it does not raise blood sugar levels is because of its high fructose content. Agave is higher in fructose than the much maligned corn syrup, and it is not easily metabolized. Overconsumption of fructose can lead to type 2 diabetes, heart disease, nonalcoholic fatty liver disease, and cancer. Although agave nectar is sweeter than sugar or honey, and so you use less, it also contains a lot of calories, so it is of little use to dieters. You are probably better off using sugar.

Molasses and Maple Syrup

Molasses is the by-product of refining sugar cane to produce sugar crystals. Until the end of World War I when the price of refined sugar dropped dramatically, it was America's sweetener of choice. Maple syrup is tapped from sugar and black maple trees. Americans have been using maple syrup to sweeten all kinds of dishes since Colonial Times, when Native Americans showed the settlers how to tap the sap from trees. Molasses is full of vitamins and minerals (B6, magnesium, manganese, and potassium). Maple syrup is relatively low in fructose. Both are high in calories and both have distinctive tastes. Molasses is thickly bittersweet, and maple syrup tastes exactly like what you are probably used to pouring over your Sunday pancakes.

Stevia

A promising sweetener that has recently become widely available in the US is stevia. Also known as sweetleaf, stevia is extracted from the leaves of an herb native to Paraguay and Brazil. Advocates point to the fact that although it is 150 to 400 times sweeter than sugar (claims vary), it contains no calories and has a glycemic index of zero.

One reason stevia has not been used more often in the food industry is that it was kept off the US market by non-nutritive sweetener lobbyists who persuaded the FDA to ban the competition. A few years ago, the European Union approved this natural sweetener as a sugar substitute, and the US soon followed suit.

Now stevia is grown in the US, mostly in California, as well as in other countries around the world, Japan being a major producer. You can even find the live plants for sale at your gardening center and in seed catalogs if you are interested in growing your own.

You may wonder why, even with the ban being lifted, the food industry and consumers still have not warmly embraced stevia. Besides the time it takes for consumers to hear about it and try it for themselves and then decide to like it, stevia may be more or less another case of "too good to be true." One problem is that although it tastes sweet initially, after a few bites the sweetness does not retain the same staying power as sugar. Others claim that some stevia brands have a lingering acrid taste. When used in cooking, stevia can turn some dishes an unappetizing brown color. Makers of stevia have been working on these issues, so in the next couple of years these glitches will probably be resolved.

If you are interested in giving sweetleaf a try, many consumers agree that the Trader Joe's brand seems to taste better than most. The Truvía brand is also popular. One difference between stevia and processed sugar is that the granules seem more powdery. Stevia certainly dissolves in hot or cold tea as rapidly as processed sugar and better than the other sweeteners mentioned.

Other Herbal Sweeteners

If none of the above options appeal to you, you can try sweetening your tea naturally with botanicals. Classic choices include cardamom, cinnamon, elderberry flowers, hibiscus flowers, licorice root, dried orange and tangerine peels, and sliced fruit such as blueberries, strawberries, or apples. Your tea will not taste sugary sweet, and you will add a new dimension. Remember you can always scent your tea, too.

Lemon and Milk

Lemon goes well with black or green China teas and can improve the flavor of some herbal teas markedly. No matter which tea you choose to drink with lemon, remember that a little goes a long way, and a lot of lemon is as overpowering as adding too much salt to a dish. The sweet-sour citrus taste of lemon is due to the proportion of citric acid and natural sugar in the fruit. Immature fruit will be more acidic. The sweeter taste evolves as the fruit matures and continues to ripen after it is picked. To gauge the sweetness of a lemon or lime, pick it up in your hand and gently roll it between your fingers. The skin will give somewhat and you will feel the juice inside. If the skin is rock-hard, the fruit is not yet ripe.

If you enjoy adding milk to your tea, know that it tastes especially good in classic robust black teas such as Assam, Ceylon, English breakfast, or Irish breakfast. Many tea lovers will tell you that milk does not taste as good in green and white teas. However, milk provides added calcium and vitamin D. When it comes to additives, it is advised not to add both milk and lemon to your tea or the milk will curdle in the hot water.

How to Prepare Medicinal Herbal Teas

Medicinal brews probably have been concocted ever since humans walked the earth. Medicinal infusions and decoctions take longer to make than a beverage tea, but many alternative health practitioners insist that they are worth the effort of choosing a collection of fresh herbs, cleaning and chopping them, and bruising the roots and seeds. Herbalists claim that most commercial herbal teabags lack the brightness, verve, and strength of high-quality fresh or dried botanicals. Consequently, the therapeutic action of your own preparations is probably better than buying an herbal teabag.

You already have been brewing herbal infusions for enjoyment by steeping herbs for up to five minutes. This generates a light, palatable tisane. For beverage infusions, you do not necessarily bring the water to a rolling boil nor pay strict attention to an exact brewing time; you simply infuse for taste.

With medicinal infusions, things work slightly differently. First, you usually use only the flowers, leaves, and soft stems. Always boil the water (approximately one teaspoon dried or one tablespoon of fresh herbs to one cup of water) before pouring it over the ingredients, and cover the brew while steeping. This ensures that the essential oils, which contain many of the healthful ingredients, do not evaporate. Steeping time is ten to fifteen minutes, which results in a more concentrated, bitter infusion than for a beverage herbal tea. Always steep in an enamel, nonmetal, or stainless steel teapot.

Strain away the plant material, and your drink is ready to be taken hot immediately or cold later. The average dose is two to four cups per day, depending on the affliction you wish to affect. Infusions are often ingested to flush toxins from the system or to cool body temperature by inducing a sweat. To preserve the nutrients and not let the infusion spoil, place the preparation in a lidded-glass container and store in the refrigerator for up to a few days. If you need to drink the infusion hot to bring down a fever for example, you can steep and store it in a thermos. As the thermos is airtight, it will keep the infusion hot for several hours.

Cold Infusions

Herbalists prepare an infusion in cold water when they wish to extract the essence from a mucilaginous plant or when the essential oil to be extracted is quite volatile. The term "mucilaginous" means that the nutritive part of the plant to be extracted is slimy or gummy. Althea root (marshmallow root) and flaxseed are examples. Rather than make a decoction from roots, some herbalists prepare a cold infusion, especially if the product is to be applied externally.

To put together a cold infusion, lightly pack the botanical(s) into a lidded, nonmetal container like a quart jar and fill it with cold water. Refrigerate overnight. In the morning, pour the liquid through a sieve and discard the plant matter. Your cold infusion is ready to use.

Decoctions

Herbalists generally prepare decoctions from the tougher materials of the plants, those parts that do not give up their essential oils easily. Usually you will make a decoction from the roots, barks, large seeds, and/or berries, or when you want to extract the maximum amount of essential oils from lighter materials.

Before you begin, you might want to bruise or mash the materials using a mortar and pestle to facilitate the release of the essential oils. In an enamel, nonmetal or stainless steel pot, bring the water to a rolling boil. Use one tablespoon of seeds and berries or one-half ounce of dried roots to two cups of water. After the water reaches a rolling boil, add the plant materials, cover, and simmer gently for twenty minutes to one hour. At the end of the process, approximately half of the water will be lost, so it is customary to add enough cold water to make up the original volume.

Because decoctions take more time and effort to produce, typically enough is made to store in the refrigerator in a lidded glass container. The brew will remain stable for at least one week.

Infusions and decoctions can be prepared from single plants or from more than one, three being a round number of plants that many herbalists like to use. You can even mix together both types of preparations. To accomplish this task, prepare the decoction, and add the lighter materials during the last ten to fifteen minutes of steeping time. Decoctions are stronger than infusions, so to diffuse the bitter taste put one to two tablespoons of the liquid in the cup and fill the rest with hot or cold water.

How to Brew a Beverage Herbal Tea

There are many ways to brew a superior-tasting herbal beverage. Here is one method. Start with one cup of natural, filtered tap water. You might want to boil the water, although some herbalists recommend you do not let the water reach the boiling point. If it does, cool it for a minute or two before adding the herbs. If you live at an altitude above 5,000 feet where water boils at a lower temperature, boiling or not boiling the water probably does not make a difference as to the taste and health benefits of the finished brew.

While the water is heating, chop one teaspoon of fresh leaves, tender stems, flowers, and/or crushed seeds. A variety of fresh herbs is not always available, especially in winter, so you can measure one-half teaspoon of dried leaves, either single botanicals or combinations. A half teaspoon of dried botanicals equals one teaspoon of fresh herb. Place the material in a nonmetal container.

When the water is ready, pour it over the herbs and cover the container with a lid. This keeps important essential oils from evaporating. Steep the brew for no more than five minutes. Finally, strain the tisane either through a piece of cheesecloth, mesh, or a coffee filter (metal tea strainers do not always retain every bit of herb), and pour the liquid into a teacup. If you care for sweetener, add sugar, honey, agave, or stevia now. Stir once, and drink while hot.

Eight

Where to Find Tea

This chapter discusses where to find tea and herbal teas. It lists Internet resources that can be used as tea guides, some of which illustrate what the different types of tea look like. It also addresses how to grow your own herbal tea garden and lists twenty common botanicals to grow for herbal tea use.

To find loose leaf and herbal teas, check out your local health food store. Look in your area for coffee and tea shops that sell loose leaf tea. Explore your local neighborhoods.

There are various tea companies that specialize in online sales of loose leaf tea. Some of the more popular online tea sellers are www.mightyleaf.com, www.adagio.com, www.culinaryteas.com, www.artoftea.com, www.teavana.

com, www.englishteastore.com, and www.ezentea.com. All of these websites depict tea in its dry form, and sometimes brewed. As with any online shopping, pay attention to customer reviews.

There are also tea rooms and houses, and if you like their tea, you might ask where they get their tea and how you can purchase some. Wherever you go to buy tea, it is recommended that you buy loose tea and buy organic. You can be sure that loose tea is not put together from fannings and dust, and so it has the best flavor and most nutrients. As with food, organic teas have a better chance of not containing chemicals and hormones that you probably would not want to imbibe. Because organic fertilizers are certified organic, the tea will retain more and better quality nutrients as well.

Going to a place that sells loose leaf tea can be very overwhelming. Here is a suggestion for what to do. When you visit a tea shop or purchase a tea online, you will notice that loose leaf tea is sold by the ounce. You only need one teaspoonful of tea per cup, sometimes less, depending on your individual taste. According to the website www.youmeandtea.com, one ounce of tea provides eight to fourteen cups of tea. The reason for the variation is because some teas are lighter in weight than others, so you get more or less of an amount of tea per ounce. Also you may prefer to brew your tea light, medium, or strong, and some consumers will want to do a second potting or more. It is recommended that you purchase only a small amount at first (such as an ounce) to try and see if you like it, and then reorder in a larger quantity.

Internet Resources

Here is a list of websites that you can use as good references to illustrate what the different types of tea look like. They also refer to studies on health and give brewing tips.

- **www.ageless.co.za**—This website gives descriptive, medicinal, and infusion information on dozens of herbs from aconite to ylang ylang.

- **www.amolis.com/treatment/health-guide**—This commercial site also gives valuable information on teas and infusions to treat diseases. Information is offered on the history of the plant, its medicinal uses and treatments, and sites that discuss effectiveness studies.

- **www.artoftea.com/learn_about_tea**—This site out of Beverly Hills, California, teaches about all varieties of teas and how they relate to Ayurvedic medicine.

- **http://blog/espemporium.com/post/What-Are-The-Largest-Tea-Producing-Countries-In-The-World.aspx**—This blog site gives the latest available data on tea-producing countries.

- www.brassicatea.com—This site relates the origin, production methods, and health benefits of Brassica tea.

- http://bristen.com/teasChart.htm—This website details a chart of the names, Latin names, and healing properties of a variety of herbs for infusion. This general site also has a gardeners' journal and talks about cooking with herbs.

- www.catteacprner.com/teadigest.htm—*Tea Digest* is all about tea for the consumer online.

- www.celestialseasonings.com—This site sells tea and presents valuable information about teas and herbal tea combinations for health and well-being.

- www.coffeetea.about.com/library/weekly—This website covers the latest information about all kinds of tea, tea accoutrements, and cultural aspects of tea (and coffee).

- www.enjoyingtea.com—This website focuses on everything tea, including health benefits and recipes.

- www.freshcup.com—*Fresh Cup Magazine* is a magazine for tea and coffee professionals. It includes updated material on tea drinking for healthy living, among other topics.

- **www.houdeasianart.com**—*The Art of Tea.* This monthly, started in 2007, focuses on Chinese tea.

- **www.inpursuitoftea.com**—This website is mostly devoted to Asian or Eastern tea, including brewing, cultural traditions, and information on herbal infusions.

- **www.LIVESTRONG.com**—This website covers various aspects of health, including teas and herbal teas. It offers descriptions, uses, precautions, and quotes from recent research studies, giving annotated data. It is a valuable site for herb and tea enthusiasts, and was used as an important source for this book.

- **www.miyerbamate.com**—This website is devoted to all aspects of yerba mate brews, including health benefits and cultural traditions.

- **www.nutraingredients-usa.com**—This website releases breaking news on supplements and nutrition in North America, including articles related to black tea, green tea, white tea, and herbal teas.

- **www.teamag.com**—This online magazine is devoted to tea.

- www.teamuse.com—This website has articles on different aspects of tea, including history and culture, the state of the industry, and tea chemistry.

- www.teatimemagazine.com—*Tea Time Magazine* covers a wide range of tea subjects.

- www.teausa.com—This is the official website of The Tea Association of the USA, Specialty Tea Institute, and Tea Council USA. It offers the latest information on the state of the industry. It also relates facts on tea, tea and health, and brewing tips. This site served as an important source for writing this book.

- www.teaviews.com—*Tea Time Gazette* is an international newsletter devoted to tea.

- www.theherbarium.wordpress.com/ category/3-internal-herbal-medicines/1- infusions-decoctions—This website gives detailed instructions on medicinal infusions and decoctions of herbs and teas.

- www.the-leaf.org—This is an interactive online tea magazine.

- www.therepublicoftea.com/Tea-101—This educational email series offered by The Republic of Tea covers tea varieties, blends, origins, the art of steeping and herbal infusions, therapeutic benefits, and more. It also sells tea.

- www.TheTeaHouseTimes.com—This bi-monthly print and online magazine explores teahouses plus up-to-date information on tea.

- www.umm.edu/altmed/articles—The University of Maryland Medical Center's website shows the results of research they perform on tea and herbs. Type in the botanical you want in the Search column and data about health benefits, risks, and recent research will come up. This site was used as an important source for writing this book.

- www.webmd.com—This is a website with descriptive and medical information on herbs and tea. It gives names, description, medicinal properties, side effects, possible drug interactions, and dosage. This is an excellent site that was used as an important source for writing this book.

- www.wtea.com/about-tea_health-benefits.aspx—This website is devoted to tea's health benefits, among other tea-related topics.

Where to Get Herbs

Herbal tea drinkers who want to make their own blends or drink a single ingredient tea often purchase their ingredients at natural food stores that offer herbs conveniently dried, pre-cut, and sifted in amounts that are more than a person usually can cultivate in the garden and/or which do not grow in all climates.

Other tea drinkers will prefer to gather their own herbs in the wild for freshness. Unfortunately, many herbalists do not recommend gathering herbs in the wild for making infusions unless you know for sure that the area has not been sprayed with pesticides or herbicides. People may think that they can go to the local playground and pick some dandelions, but this is not always the case, as those areas are often sprayed to eradicate weeds and insects.

Nowadays, too, there is the alarming GMO (genetically modified organism) problem to contend with. The effects of these genetically altered crops do not stay within the confines of their fields. They spread potentially dangerous and unalterable modifications far and wide by wind and runoff. GMOs can change the internal structure of an herb forever. Such changes have the potential to destroy the beneficial characteristics of the plant. The sad truth is even in the wild, truly organic organisms may soon cease to exist.

If you still wish to gather plant-based edibles on your own, here are some tips:

- Do not take plants from the roadside, as they are most exposed to pesticides, herbicides, car emissions, and other pollutants.

- Pick before 10 am, when the essential oils are most concentrated in the flowers and leaves; these are usually the parts you will harvest.

- Do not take more than one-third of the plant to give it an opportunity to regenerate.

- As soon as you arrive home, rinse the material thoroughly in cold water to remove dust and clinging dirt.

- Try not to bruise or tear the delicate leaves and flowers so they do not lose their essential oils.

- If you are not going to drink the tea fresh, tie the botanicals in bunches and hang them upside down from the ceiling in a cool, dry, dark place with good circulation.

- Tie fairly small bunches. Big ones tend to cut off air circulation and causes mold on the plant.

- Dried herbs tend to look alike, so be sure to label each bunch. Buy tie-on labels like those used for pricing clothing at garage sales.

- After the botanicals dry thoroughly, remove leaves and flowers from the stems and crush the leaves. Keep flowers whole and dice stems and roots if you want to use them, too. Throw away woody stems; they have few nutrients and do not taste good.

- Place each plant part in a separate airtight container. For example, do not put dandelion leaves and roots in the same jar, as each has a distinctive flavor and is sometimes used for a different reason.

- Store your containers in a cool place away from the light.

Growing Your Own Herbal Tea Garden

Perhaps you cannot find a reliable supplier, or maybe you yearn to understand the herbs you incorporate into your body at a more fundamental and profound level. If this description fits, you are a likely candidate to grow your own herbal tea garden. After all, people have been growing herbs in pretty much the same simple ways for centuries.

Advantages of cultivating your own are that you will know exactly where your herbs come from and they will be as fresh as possible. Also herbs are one of the few "crops" that have never been genetically modified. There are too many of them and they grow everywhere and probably modification does not pay the big producers. So when you drink an herbal tea, basically you are drinking the same product with more or less the same taste with the same nutrients your ancestors enjoyed. This makes herbal teas great choices for better health.

Gardening is doubly healthy for you because it gives you a good physical workout. An herb garden is also bound to attract beneficial insects and pollinators to the rest of your yard and keep it in the pink along with your body. If you live in an apartment or do not have space to plant an herb garden, hints on how to create a kitchen window garden will be offered later in this chapter.

Laying Out an Herb Garden

Botanical gardens have formed part of the landscape since the Middle Ages, and probably before that time, too. The earliest documented herb garden plan is from a ninth-century Benedictine monastery. In those days and into the Renaissance and beyond, gardeners planted botanicals in more or less separate areas devoted to herbs for seasoning, medicine, fragrance, dyeing, and fiber. Each garden was walled by a number of methods to ward off pests and create an intimate, sheltered spot to delight the senses. The medicinal garden often consisted of raised beds laid out in rectangles or squares with brick or gravel pathways in between to make caring for the plants and harvesting easier. Each bed housed a single plant. As time went on, more elaborate designs were created, including a series of complicated knots, spirals, and the like.

You do not need to go to a lot of trouble to create a useful, enjoyable herbal tea garden. The idea of a single species in each raised bed is a good one because many herbs such as borage and the mints are notorious spreaders that will take over the garden if you are not vigilant about keeping them confined.

Here is a simple, effective design: Arrange four 4-by-4 raised beds in a block around a central circle. Inside the circle you can plant a strawberry pyramid, or a bush like a rose or rosemary. Construct little pathways between the beds with pebbles or bricks. In the square beds plant four of your favorite herbs in rich, organic soil. Water thoroughly and regularly and keep the garden weed-free.

If you are ambitious, you might want to extend a long rectangular bed across the back of the garden and plant taller herbs or bushes. Make sure the back border is on the north side so that the taller plants do not shade the low-growing ones in front of them.

To add variety, position at convenient locations some pot herbs such as basil, dill, parsley, or even a real tea plant; that is, a *Camellia sinensis*. Remember that you will need to move your tea plant inside for the winter unless you live in a tropical or semi-tropical climate. Potted tea plants do well as long as the soil is kept well-drained and you mist them frequently.

If you like to travel and are looking for inspiration on growing an herb garden, there are three famous gardens that are often recommended by herbalists and tea lovers alike. Although the Japanese Garden in Portland, Oregon is magnificent, it is too grandiose to act as a model for a humble home herbarium. Instead, go to the Lan Su Chinese Garden. It is located in the heart of Portland's Chinatown (239 Northwest Everett Street, Portland, Oregon 97209). The garden with its teahouse, pond, and other buildings covers only one city block, but once inside, you will think you stepped into the house and grounds of a secluded Chinese country estate.

Second on the list is the Chelsea Physic Garden, a walled herb garden tucked away in the heart of the Chelsea borough of London, just steps from the busy King's Road and the Thames Embankment. The garden was founded in 1673 by the Worshipful Society of Apothecaries for its apprentices to study the medicinal qualities of plants. This gem of an old-fashioned herb garden is located at 66 Royal Hospital Road, London, SW3, England.

Last, and perhaps a favorite of many, are The Cloisters, a branch of the New York Metropolitan Museum, located in Fort Tryon Park on the north end of the island of Manhattan. The Cloisters are dedicated to the art and architecture of medieval Europe. The area includes four herb gardens laid out in true medieval fashion with hundreds of plants, most of them used during the Middle Ages. Do not miss the espaliered pear tree that has been trained to grow on a trellis. This makes a great way to plant a bush for herbal infusions if you have limited space.

It goes without saying that when you visit different tea gardens, you are not allowed to pick your own herbs from the gardens. Some of these gardens, however, occasionally have herbs/plants for sale in the gift shop area.

Indoor Tea Herb Gardening

If you cannot have an outdoor herbal tea garden, you can garden indoors. Even people who live in cold winter climates can always bring some potted herbs inside to place on a sunny window ledge to enjoy fresh herbal infusions year round. Even better news is that the *Camellia sinensis*, the true tea plant, does well in a large pot because it prefers filtered light like the kind you get indoors. Tea plants also prefer rich, well-drained soil.

For any herb/plant that you bring indoors for the winter, you need to help acclimatize it to the indoor climate. Prune by removing dead leaves and branches up to one-third of the plant. Any more than that and you risk killing the plant. Wash off thoroughly any aphids or other pests clinging to the branches and leaves. Keep the plant away from drafts and heat blasting from your radiators. You will always lose some leaves, but the plant should remain healthy.

If you have several small windows, an ideal way to garden is to plant each herb in a separate flower pot with drainage holes. Cover the holes with a single layer of cheesecloth or a coffee filter so that soil does not work its way out through the bottom. Set each pot in a saucer and put the saucer on top of a metal trivet on the window ledge. That way, you do not leave water stains on the sill. If you are handy with a hammer and saw, you can build your own narrow rectangular container from wood or metal to fit your window precisely, and plant more than one herb in it.

Fill your containers with a mixture of organic potting soil and planting compost. Some indoor gardeners prefer to buy small container plants at a garden center instead of sewing seeds because they do not want plants to germinate all over the place and intermingle. Rotate the flowerpots or turn the window box around every couple of weeks so the plants will grow straight and strong. You will harvest leaves as you need them, but for window gardens, it is essential to keep the plants clipped back so they do not grow into each other.

Most herbs are comfortable with good soil that is not too rich. Lavender, for example, actually thrives best in poor quality soil. You only need to fertilize once a month or so whether the botanicals are planted in the house or outdoors. Here is another tip. Whenever you water, mist under the leaves to discourage aphids, spider mites, whitefly, and other pests. If your plants are in fairly small containers, you can give them a monthly treat by bathing them in the kitchen sink with the sprayer.

Twenty Easy-to-Grow Tea Garden Botanicals

Following are descriptions of twenty herbal botanicals that have been cultivated for centuries to make beverage and medicinal teas. They all flourish just about anywhere in the US. Once established, you will have a hard time killing them off. Rose bushes are the exception; as queens of the garden, they can be finicky. One type that survives just about anywhere and that puts up with all sorts of abuse is the wild rose, also known as the dog rose.

In the following list, you will see listed the botanical's height so you know whether to plant it at the back of the garden, in the middle or as a border. Useful information, such as flower colors for aesthetic reasons, parts used in herbal medicine, how the botanical tastes in a tea, and other tips are also given.

Angelica—perennial or biennial; height: 3–6 feet; exposure: prefers partial shade; soil: moist rich, slightly acidic; flowers: greenish-white honey-scented flowers that look like umbrellas; parts used: leaves, seeds, roots; taste: celery-like.

Borage—an annual, but it reseeds so readily it can be considered a perennial; height: 1–3 feet; exposure: sun to partial shade; soil: fairly dry; flowers: nodding clusters of flowers that look like little blue stars and attract hoards of bees; parts used: leaves and flowers; taste: cucumber-like. Note: Borage proliferates madly, so sowing it in a raised bed is strongly advised. This plant tolerates poor soil conditions well.

Calendula—annual, but the flower heads produce so many seeds, all you need do is save them to sow the following season; height: 6 inches to 3 feet; exposure: full sun; soil: average; flowers: bright orange, parts used: flowers; taste: saffron-like, slightly bitter. Note: Only the small, orange-flowered calendula (pot marigold) is used in herbal medicine. Plant marigolds as borders because of their short height and also because they repel nematodes and other pests.

Chamomile—perennial; height: 3 inches to 1 foot; exposure: sun to partial shade; soil: well-drained; flowers: daisy-like with yellow centers and silvery white petals; parts used: flowers; taste: apple-like.

Chrysanthemum—perennial: height: 1–5 feet; exposure: full to partial sun; soil: sandy and rich; flowers: daisy-like white or yellow disc florets; parts used: flower; taste: artichoke-like, aromatic. Note: Before horticulturalists started creating different varieties, all chrysanthemums used to have button-like, white and yellow flowers. These are still the kind the Chinese use today to scent tea.

(Red) Clover—perennial; height: 2 feet; exposure: sun; soil: average to fertile, neutral to alkaline; flowers: pinkish-purple flower heads; parts used: dried blossoms; taste: sweet.

Fennel—perennial; height: 3–5 feet; exposure: sun; soil: lime-rich garden soil; flowers: flat, yellow, umbelliferous; parts used: seeds; taste: licorice-like. Note: Pick the seeds before they have time to scatter unless you want to raise hundreds of little fennel plants.

Lavender—perennial; height: 2–3 feet; exposure: sun; soil: dry, chalky; flowers: purple spikes; parts used: flowers; taste: clean, aromatic. Trim off the dead spikes to keep the plant healthy and encourage more blooms.

Lemon balm—perennial; height: 2–4 feet; exposure: sun to partial shade, but some of my plants do okay in a lot of shade; soil: average—this plant is not picky; flowers: tiny white flowers along the stems display modest blooms, but the leaf fragrance is reminiscent of lemon sherbet; parts used: leaf; taste: lemon-like, refreshing.

Marjoram—perennial; height: 1–2 feet; exposure: sun to partial shade; soil: light, but moist and alkaline; flowers: clusters of small, pale white or red blooms that grow on spikes; parts used: leaves; taste: oregano-like with hints of sweetness and warmth.

Mint—perennial; height: 18 inches to 4 feet, depending on species; exposure: partial to full shade; soil: any type, but prefers moist; flowers: depending on the variety, small, unremarkable, white, purple or violet grow at the top of spikes; parts used: leaves; taste: depending on the variety, peppermint, orangey, lemony, pineapple-like, spearmint, apple minty, chocolate minty. Note: All varieties taste minty and refreshing, some have fruity overtones. The newer leaves concentrate more of the flavor. Be sure to plant mints in raised beds because they spread rapidly and are difficult to control once established.

Monarda (also known as bergamot, bee balm, and oswego tea)—perennial; height: 1–3 feet, tends to spread horizontally (at least mine does); exposure: sun to partial shade; soil: moist (but not too wet), acidic; flowers: pretty, two-lipped scarlet, pink, violet, or white blossoms; parts used: leaves and flowers; taste: citrus-minty. Note: If you want to approximate the taste of Earl Grey tea by making your own, add some of the leaves to China black or Darjeeling.

Nettle—perennial; height: 1–8 feet, though I have never seen it grow so tall; exposure: sun; soil: moist and rich in organic matter; flowers: clusters of small, greenish blossoms; parts used: dried leaves; taste: tasteless, but can be perked up by adding mint or citrus peels. Note: Please be cautious around nettles. The hairs on the leaves contain formic acid, which stings and blisters the skin horribly. The dried leaves are harmless.

Parsley—biennial; height: no more than a foot; exposure: partial to full shade; soil: rich, moist; flowers: greenish-yellow or white; parts used: leaves; taste: no surprise here, it is parsley-like, which means cool and refreshing. Note: Parsley makes a good kitchen window container plant because of its contained habit. Harvest the leaves before the plant blooms.

Rose—perennial in most places, though I lose a
bush or two every year here in Colorado, where
temperatures can plummet; height: depending on
the variety, several inches to several feet; exposure:
full sun; soil: well-drained and enriched; flowers:
stunningly beautiful often fragrant blooms in just
about every shade imaginable, although pink, red,
yellow, and white are most common; parts used:
petals and rosehips, the round fruit that develops
from spent flower blossoms; taste: the hips are
tangy and aromatic, the petals taste delicate and
flowery. Note: Roses are especially susceptible to
aphids. You do not want to use a commercial spray
on them or you will not be able to drink them
in a tea. Organic gardeners recommend using
an organic insecticidal soap or pyrethrum spray
that is based on chrysanthemums. If you have
only a couple of bushes and do not mind tedious
work, you can remove the aphids using dampened
cotton balls or cloths. Let your bushes blossom
in late spring and early summer. Deadhead them
for the petals and to produce more flowers for tea
until mid-summer. After that, let the flowers die
naturally. In time, dark red hips will form. Not all
roses bloom more than once during a season. If
you do not have repeat bloomers, leave half of the
blossoms on the bush to form healthy hips for teas.

Sage—perennial; height: 2–4 feet; exposure: sun to
partial shade; soil: dry or sandy, limy; flowers:
purple or blue blooms that form on tall spikes;
parts used: leaves; taste: somewhat like camphor,
aromatic, slightly bitter and reminiscent of poultry
seasoning, which is partly composed of sage.

Strawberry—perennial; height: 6–10 inches; exposure:
full sun, although my plants do well in partial
shade; soil: rich, moist, well-drained; flowers:
five-petal white flowers with yellow centers that
transform into fat, juicy red strawberry fruit;
parts used: leaves, although herbal tea drinkers
sometimes add slices of fruit as a garnish in the
teacup; taste: slightly strawberry-like, but adding
the fresh fruit slices helps augment the flavor.

Thyme—perennial; height: 2–12 inches, depending
on the variety; exposure: sun; soil: dry and lime;
flowers: various shades of purple that are a magnet
for bees; parts used: leaves; taste: pungent, and in
my opinion, not very pleasant, but can be improved
by adding lemon balm or lemon verbena. Note:
This is a good plant for kitchen containers and it
possesses many medicinal virtues. Common thyme,
which grows to around 8" tall, is the best-tasting
for tea, although all thymes taste highly balsamic.
Many herbal tea drinkers prefer the lemon thyme
variety, which grows to 1 foot, and so is best suited

to the outdoor garden. The leaves are an antiseptic. They also keep a person from having muscle and coughing spasms, help expel gas from the digestive tract, helps a cough sufferer cough up phlegm, and helps bring down a fever. Drink a decoction to remove intestinal worms. Externally, the tea is used to rid a person of lice, crabs, parasites, and fungal infections like athletes' foot.

Valerian or garden heliotrope—perennial; height: 4 feet; exposure: sun to partial shade; soil: heavy and moist, and the plant does not mind clay; flowers: clusters of lavender, blue or pink blooms appear on the ends of long stems; part used: root; taste: strong, but soothing. Harvest the root in the fall, and leave some to regenerate the following year.

Yarrow—perennial; height: 3 feet; exposure: full sun; soil: likes fairly poor soil and is drought-tolerant; flowers: large clusters of mainly yellow or cream-colored flowers, although there is also a red-flowered variety called "paprika"; parts used: leaves and flowers; taste: astringent, sagelike. Note: Be careful with yarrow as it spreads readily through the garden and once established is hard to eradicate.

Appendix

This appendix consists of common complaints and six herbal teas to support them. More botanicals and complaints are listed in chapter 6.

Herbal Teas for Common Complaints

Arthritis and Joint Pain—burdock root, devil's claw root, flaxseed, licorice, nettles, turmeric

Bladder Infection—buchu, corn silk, couch grass, cranberry, dandelion root and leaf, parsley

Colds—ginger root, hibiscus flower, lemon balm, licorice root, red root, rosehips, thyme

Constipation—burdock root, ginger root, fennel, lemon peel, licorice root, strawberry leaves; senna leaf tea can be used sparingly, but be aware that it has a very strong laxative effect

Cough—elecampane, red clover, coltsfoot, ginger root, horehound, althea root

Diarrhea—agrimony, blackberry or raspberry hip, chamomile, cinnamon, licorice root, spearmint

Fatigue—dandelion root, ginseng, licorice, peppermint, rosemary, sage

Fever—catnip, borage, elderflower, feverfew, lovage, yarrow

Headache—ginger, lavender, lemon balm, peppermint, rosemary, spearmint

Hemorrhage—alfalfa, blackberry, goldenseal, lady's mantle, nettle, yarrow

Indigestion/Heartburn/Gas—angelica, chamomile, fennel, ginger, peppermint, spearmint

Inflammation—basil, cardamom, celery seed, ginger, parsley, rooibos, turmeric

Insomnia—catnip, chamomile, hops, passionflower, St. John's wort, valerian

Liver Tonic—burdock root, dandelion root, kelp, milk thistle, nettle, rosehips

Nausea—angelica, chamomile, ginger, lavender, lemon verbena, raspberry hip

Skin Problems—chamomile, dandelion leaf, hibiscus, oat straw, rooibos, rosehips

Sore Throat—althea root, borage, honeysuckle flowers, lavender, sage, slippery elm; honeysuckle flowers are difficult to find unless you have your own honeysuckle vine and it is in flower; they are available at Chinese food stores

Stress—hops, lavender, lemon verbena, linden, rosehips and petals, skullcap

Toothache—calendula, clove, lavender, lemon balm, peppermint, spearmint

Weight Loss—alfalfa, cinnamon, fennel, guaraná, honeybush, vanilla

To discover which flavors you like best and how the substances interact with your body, first try them as "singles," then as "doubles," and so on, adding one herb at a time. Then try experimenting with the ratios until you find what best suits you.

For example, to make a tea to mitigate stress, you might buy some dried lemon balm leaves, hops flowers, feverfew flowers, licorice powder, rosehips, and skullcap at your local organic grocery. Make separate infusions from 1 teaspoon of each botanical. Next, mix together ½ teaspoon lemon balm and ½ teaspoon hops, and decide how you like this tisane. Another time, blend an infusion from ½ teaspoon lemon balm, ¼ teaspoon feverfew and ¼ teaspoon hops, and so forth.

Your final recipe might consist of ½ teaspoon lemon balm, ¼ teaspoon feverfew, ⅛ teaspoon hops, ⅛ teaspoon crushed rosehips and a dash or two of licorice powder. Or you may prefer lemon balm exclusively with a dash of licorice powder to awaken the lemony taste. Then again, perhaps you will be bowled over by one of the other single herbs.

Recipes

"Blow Away That Cold" Herbal Tea

2 teaspoons raspberry leaves and hips

1 teaspoon feverfew flowers

½ teaspoon fresh, grated ginger root

Brew as an herbal infusion.

Chamomile Tea

To prepare a fresh chamomile herbal tea, steep 1 table-spoon of the fresh flowers (or 2 teaspoons of dried) in one cup boiling water for five to ten minutes.

Clove Tea

To make your own strong decoction of clove tea, boil 3 ounces of the chopped root in a pint of water for one-half hour. Sieve away the root, and you will have a medicinal-strength brew.

Flaxseed Tea

The taste of this infusion is soothing and gelatinous. When preparing flaxseed for an herbal tea, it is suggested that you first grind the seeds. Then add 2 teaspoons to 1 cup of boiling water and allow to steep for at least ten minutes before drinking.

Gingko Tea

Herbalists recommend using 1 teaspoon per cup of boiling water. Infuse for 10 minutes until the brew turns yellow. Strain and drink.

Honeybush Tea

Prepare honeybush tea by boiling 2 to 3 tablespoons in a quart of water for twenty minutes. Strain and serve. Africans drink both honeybush and rooibos with sugar and milk, but the infusion tastes equally good without any additives. Store leftovers in the refrigerator for a sweet, sugar-free iced tea.

Irish Moss Tonic

To make an Irish moss tonic combine ½ ounce of the dried seaweed with ½ ounce cocoa, and boil in 1 pint milk and 1 pint water for ten to fifteen minutes. Strain and season with licorice or cinnamon and sweeten with honey. This type of herbal preparation falls under the category of "white infusions" in color healing.

Lavender Rose Tea

Following is a recipe that takes advantage of the light flavor of rose petals in combination with the clean taste of lavender.

½ cup Lady Grey green tea

1 tablespoon red rose petals

2 teaspoons lavender buds

½ teaspoon allspice berries, crushed

Blend ingredients well, and use ½ teaspoon per cup.

Licorice Decoction

To make your own strong decoction, boil 3 ounces of the chopped root in 1 pint of water for one-half hour. Sieve away the root, and you will have a medicinal-strength brew.

Morning Tea

You do not need to search high and low for a gourmet scented tea to enjoy a flowery brew. Simply combine edible blossoms and spices of your choice (such as rose, honeysuckle, lavender) with your favorite loose green tea. When you do this, you also reap the health benefits of the added botanicals. The following is an example.

2 teaspoons Lady Grey green tea, any brand (Two popular varieties of this tea exist. Both consist of Earl Grey tea. One variety adds lavender for a clean taste, and the other adds Seville oranges for a citrus taste.)

½ teaspoon lemon verbena leaves, fresh or dried, to
   refresh you

½ teaspoon alfalfa to give you a shot of vitamins A,
   B, C, K, and minerals

¼ teaspoon ginseng for revitalization

¼ teaspoon guaraná for energy

Pinch of safflower for stimulation (or saffron,
   although be aware that saffron is very expensive)

Mix all of the ingredients together, except for the fresh
lemon, and store in the refrigerator in an airtight jar. Depending on how strong you take your tea, this recipe will
render several cups. Some people prefer to only use ½ teaspoon per cup of hot water. Add a squirt or two of lemon
to each serving to enliven the brew.

Parsley Tea

To prepare parsley tea, chop ¼ cup of fresh leaves or measure 2 teaspoons of chopped dried leaves. Pop in a few
seeds if you are drinking the tea to counteract symptoms of
arthritis or rheumatism. Pour 1 cup of boiling water over
the leaves, steep for 5 minutes, strain away the leaves and
drink hot. Parsley can taste bitter, so you might want to
add a fresh chopped stevia leaf, honey, or even a squirt of
lemon to your brew.

Rooibos Tea

Prepare rooibos somewhat differently from other herbal teas. Use 1 to 4 teaspoons per cup of boiling water, steep for ten minutes instead of the usual five minutes, pour through a coffee filter and enjoy it plain or sweetened. In spite of using more of the herb, rooibos is economical because you can re-steep the leaves up to three times before you need to discard them. The infusion also tastes delicious iced.

Spicy Chai

1 cup Chai, brewed from a Chai teabag in milk

½ teaspoon kelp, a nutrient that cleanses arteries and the reproductive system, increases vitality, and is a remedy for eczema, asthma, anemia, headache, and goiter

¼ teaspoon cinnamon, ground

¼ teaspoon green or black cardamom pod, crushed

Blend all ingredients and stir with a licorice or cinnamon stick.

Vanilla Milk Tea

If you go the decaffeinated route, you can also serve this to children.

4 cups soft, filtered water

2 cups whole milk

1 tablespoon White Peony tea

2 teaspoons vanilla extract

Honey (or stevia) to taste

Boil the water. Meanwhile, in a separate pot, bring the milk to a simmer and add sweetener. When the water has boiled, add the tea and steep in a covered nonmetal container for five minutes. Sieve away the tea leaves and add the sweetened milk and extract. Stir well and pour into cups. Serves six.

Russian Tea

Russian tea is a full-bodied black tea brewed strongly in a samovar, a metal urn. Traditionally, the water is heated by passing a tube filled with hot charcoal through the hollow center. These days, most samovars are energized by little propane units that fit into the bottom like in chafing dishes. However, you don't need a samovar to brew a fortifying pot of Russian tea. By tradition, the tea is served with lemon and sugar cubes. Russians like their tea very sweet, so they might add 1 cup sugar, which may be too sweet for most people. The natural sugars in the juices and spices in this recipe should be enough.

5 cups Russian Caravan (or Irish Breakfast) tea, strongly brewed*

½ cup orange juice, fresh squeezed

¼ cup pineapple juice

¼ cup lemon juice, fresh squeezed

1 teaspoon cinnamon pieces, crushed

1 teaspoon allspice, crushed

½ teaspoon cloves, crushed

Sugar to taste

Add the rest of the ingredients to the hot brewed tea and bring to a boil. Let mixture steep for five minutes, then pour through the strainer into a warmed teapot. The strainer will capture the leaves and bits of spices so they don't lodge in your teeth. Pour from the teapot into glass mugs. Serves six.

*Note: Brewing tea strongly means increasing the ratio of tea to water, not extending the brewing time, which can make the tea bitter and unappetizing.

Iced Green Earl Grey Tea

Here's a variation on traditional Black Earl Grey tea. Brew a cup of your favorite green tea, adding a few fresh bergamot leaves to the brew. Since you are going to add ice, you should add twice as much tea as you would if you were going to drink the tea hot. Pour over ice and enjoy. If you cannot find fresh bergamot in the store, grow your own. Since bergamot is a mint, it is easy to grow in almost any climate and spreads readily throughout the garden. This mint will also thrive in a pot in a sunny window.

Glossary

Annual—a plant that dies down completely after one season's growth. Example: basil.

Biennial—a plant that regenerates for one season, and then dies off completely. Often roots and leaves form the first year, and flowers and fruit during the second year. Example: parsley.

Brassica tea—green tea with the addition of sulforaphane (SGS), an antioxidant substance extracted from broccoli.

Camellia sinensis—Latin name for the tea plant, also known as *Thea sinensis camellia.*

Chocolate—ground and roasted cacao seeds fashioned into bars, pastes, powders, or syrups. A current trend is to flavor tea with chocolate.

Cocoa—powdered cocoa bean from which the butter fat has been removed, and therefore, it is considered healthier than chocolate. Cocoa is also added to tea to flavor it and reap health benefits.

Doctrine of Signatures—theory invented in the Middle Ages which posits that everything in the universe is interlinked and that these connections manifest in like colors, forms, and odors.

Herb—a strict definition refers to any seed plant whose stem withers and dies to the ground after each season's growth, as opposed to a tree or bush whose woody stem lives from year to year. Example: mint. Herbs are used for medicinal and culinary purposes.

Honeybush—a species of *Cyclopedia* bush, native to South Africa, from which an herbal infusion is prepared for better health and enjoyment. Honeybush contains an array of minerals and flavones, isoflavones, and xanthines, which are powerful antioxidants.

Perennial—a plant that lives for more than two years, whether or not it loses its leaves at the end of a season and then regenerates them during the following season. Some herbs are perennials, as are trees and shrubs. Examples: bee balm (a perennial herb), *Camellia sinensis* (a perennial bush).

PETE, PET—a chemical substance found in some plastic bottles and in cans that can leak carcinogens.

Rooibos—*(Aspalathus linearis)*—also known as "red tea" or "redbush tea," this fashionable herbal infusion, green-colored until it is oxidized, is a noted antioxidant said to strengthen the capillary walls.

Stevia—*(Stevia rebaudiana)*, also known as Sweet Leaf, it is a substance extracted from a native Paraguayan herb many times sweeter with sugar and which contains no calories.

Tea—an infusion made from the leaves of the *Camellia sinensis* plant. Infusions made from other botanicals are popularly known as herbal teas, but in the strictest sense they are not proper teas, rather herbal infusions or tisanes.

Tea Punch—green or black tea sweetened and flavored with fruit juices, spices, and often with wine or liquor. Tea punches were popular during the nineteenth century, and offshoots can be seen today in tea liqueurs, tea martinis, and other trendy alcoholic drinks prepared with a tea base.

Tisane—a traditional name for a drinking infusion made from botanicals other than the tea plant. They are often referred to as herbal infusions or herbal teas.

References

Alexopoulos, N. *European Journal of Cardiovascular Prevention and Rehabilitation.* June 2008; 15: 300–305.

Arab, L., D. Il'yasova. The epidemiology of tea consumption and colorectal cancer incidence. *J Nutr.* 2003; 133 (10): 3310S–3318S.

Ardlie, N. G., G. Glew, B. G. Schultz, C. J. Schwartz. Inhibition and reversal of platelet aggregation by methyl xanthines. *Thromb Diath Haemorrh.* 1967; 18: 670-673.

Arts, I. C. W., B. van de Putte, P. C. H. Hollman. Catechin contents of foods commonly consumed in the Netherlands. 2. Tea, wine, fruit juices, and chocolate milk. *Journal of Agricultural and Food Chemistry.* 2000; 48 (5): 1752–1757.

Astill, C., M. R. Birch, C. Dacombe, P. G. Humphrey, P. T. Martin. Factors affecting the caffeine and polyphenol contents of black and green tea infusions. *J Agric Food Chem.* 2001; 49 (11): 5340–5347.

August, D. A., J. Landau, D. Caputo, et al. Ingestion of green tea rapidly decreases prostaglandin E2 levels in rectal mucosa in humans. *Cancer Epidemiology, Biomarkers and Prevention.* 1999; 8 (8): 709–713.

Avisar, R., E. Avisar, D. Weinberger. Effect of coffee consumption on intraocular pressure. *Ann Pharmacother.* 2002; 36: 992–995.

Balentine, D.A., I. Pactau Robinson. Tea as a source of dietary antioxidants with a potential role in prevention of chronic diseases. G. Mazza, B. D. Oomah, eds. *Herbs, Botanicals, & Teas.* Lancaster: Technomic Publishing, 2000: 265–287.

Baliga, M.S., S. Rao. Radioprotective potential of mint: A brief review. *Journal of Cancer Research and Therapeutics.* 2010; 6: 255–262.

Bara, A.I., E. A. Barley. Caffeine for asthma. *Cochrane Database Syst Rev.* 2001; 4: CD001112.

Basch, E., S. Bent, I. Foppa, et al. Marigold *(Calendula officinalis)*: An evidence-based systematic review by the Natural Standard Research Collaboration. *J Herb Pharmacother.* 2006; 6 (3–4): 135–59.

Belza, A., S. Toubro, A. Astrup. The effect of caffeine, green tea and tyrosine on thermogenesis and energy intake. *Eur J Clin Nutr.* 2007; Epub ahead of print.

Bettuzzi, S., M. Brausi, F. Rizzi, G. Castagnetti, Peracchia G, Corti A. Chemoprevention of human prostate cancer by oral administration of green tea catechins in volunteers with high-grade prostate intraepithelial neoplasia: a preliminary report from a one-year proof-of-principle study. *Cancer Res.* 2006; 66 (2): 1234–12340.

Birks, J., J. Grimley Evans. Ginkgo biloba for cognitive impairment and dementia. *Cochrane Database Systems Review.* 2009 Jan 21; (1): CD003120.

Boehm, K., F. Borrelli, E. Ernst, et al. Green tea (Camellia sinensis) for the prevention of cancer. *Cochrane Database Systems Review.* 2009; (3): CD005004.

Borghi, L., T. Meschi, T. Schianchi, et al. Urine volume: stone risk factor and preventive measure. *Nephron.* 1999; 8 1 Suppl 1: 31–37.

Borrelli, F., R. Capasso, A. Russo, E. Ernst. Systematic review: green tea and gastrointestinal cancer risk. *Aliment Pharmacol Ther.* Mar 1, 2004; 19 (5): 497–510.

Boschmann, M., F. Thielecke. The effects of epigall-ocatechin-3-gallate on thermogenesis and fat oxidation in obese men: a pilot study. *J Am Coll Nutr.* 2007; 26 (4): 389S–395S.

Brown, A. L., J. Lane, C. Holyoak, B. Nicol, A. E. Mayes, T. Dadd. Health effects of green tea catechins in overweight and obese men: a randomised controlled cross-over trial. *Br J Nutr.* 2011 Jun 7: 1–10.

Bryan, J. *Nutrition Review.* February 2008; 66: 82–90.

Cabrera, C., R. Artacho, R. Giménez. Beneficial effects of green tea—a review. *Journal of the American College of Nutrition.* 2006; 25 (2): 79–99.

Cabrera, C., R. Giménez, M. C. López. Determination of tea components with antioxidant activity. *Journal of Agricultural and Food Chemistry.* 2003; 51 (15): 4427–4435.

Carlson, J. *Mayo Clinic Proceedings.* June 2007; 82: 725–732.

Carrillo, J. A., J. Benitez. Clinically significant pharmacokinetic interactions between dietary caffeine and medications. *Clin Pharmacokinet.* 2000; 39 (2): 127–153.

Carter, O., R. H. Dashwood, R. Wang, et al. Comparison of white tea, green tea, epigallocatechin-3-gallate, and caffeine as inhibitors of PhIP-induced colonic aberrant crypts. *Nutr Cancer.* 2007; 58 (1): 60–65.

Caturla, N., L. Funes, L. Pérez-Fons, V. Micol. A randomized, double-blinded, placebo-controlled study of the effect of a combination of lemon verbena extract and fish oil omega-3 fatty acid on joint management. *Journal of Alternative Complementary Medicine.* 2011, Nov 17 (11).

Checkoway, H., K. Powers, T. Smith-Weller, et al. Parkinson's disease risks associated with cigarette smoking, alcohol consumption, and caffeine intake. *Am J Epidemiol.* 2002; 155: 732–738.

Chedraui, P., G. San Miguel, L. Hidalgo, N. Morocho, S. Ross. Effect of Trifolium pratense-derived isoflavones on the lipid profile of postmenopausal women with increased body mass index. *Gynecol Endocrinol.* 2008 Nov; 24 (11): 620–624.

Chen, Z., M. B. Pettinger, C. Ritenbaugh, et al. Habitual tea consumption and risk of osteoporosis: a prospective study in the women's health initiative observational cohort. *Am J Epidemiol.* 2003; 158 (8): 772–781.

Chin, J. M., M. L. Merves, B. A. Goldberger, A. Sampson-Cone, E. J. Cone. Caffeine content of brewed teas. *Journal of Analytical Toxicology.* 2008; 32 (8): 702–704.

Choi, Y. T., C. H. Jung, S. R. Lee, et al. The green tea polyphenol (-)-epigallocatechin gallate attenuates beta-amyloid-induced neurotoxicity in cultured hippocampal neurons. *Life Sci.* 2001; 70: 603–614.

Chow, H. H., Y. Cai, I. A. Hakim, et al. Pharmacokinetics and safety of green tea polyphenols after multiple-dose administration of epigallocatechin gallate and polyphenon E in healthy individuals. *Clin Cancer Res.* 2003; 9 (9): 3312–3319.

Chow, H. S., Y. Cai, I. A. Hakim, et al. Pharmacokinetics and safety of green tea polyphenols after multiple-dose administration of epigallocatechin gallate and polyphenon E in healthy individuals. *Clinical Cancer Research.* 2003; 9 (9): 3312–3319.

Collins, K. *Health Talk*, on fennel; weekly column of the Am Inst for Cancer Res., April 14, 2008.

Cooper, R., D. J. Morre, D. M. Morre. Medicinal benefits of green tea: Part I. Review of noncancer health benefits. *J Altern Complement Med.* 2005; 11 (3): 521–528.

Cronin, J. R. Green tea extract stokes thermogenesis: will it replace ephedra? *Altern Comp Ther.* 2000; 6: 296–300.

Cui, Y., H. Morgenstern, S. Greenland, et al. Dietary flavonoid intake and lung cancer—a population-based case-control study. *Cancer.* 2008; 112 (10): 2241–2248.

Curhan, G. C., W. C. Willett, F. E. Speizer, M. J. Stamfer. Beverage use and risk of kidney stones in women. *Ann Intern Med.* 1998; 128: 534–540.

Devine, A., J. M. Hodgson, I. M. Dick, R. L. Prince. Tea drinking is associated with benefits on bone density in older women. *A.m J. Clin. Nutr.* 2007; 86 (4): 1243–1247.

Diepvens, K., K. R. Westerterp, M. S. Westerterp-Plantenga. Obesity and thermogenesis related to the consumption of caffeine, ephedrine, capsaicin and green tea. *Am J Physiol Regul Integr Comp Physiol.* 2007; 292 (1): R77–85.

Dudhea, Z., J. Louw, C. Muller, et al. Cyclopia maculata and cyclopedia subternata (honeybush tea) inhibits adiopogenesis in 3T3-Li pre-adipocytes. *Phytomedicine.* 2013; 20 (5): 401–408.

Dulloo, A. G., C. Duret, D. Rohrer, et al. Efficacy of a green tea extract rich in catechin polyphenols and caffeine in increasing 24-hour energy expenditure and fat oxidation in humans. *Am J Clin Nutr.* 1999; 70 (6): 1040–1045.

Elmets, C. A., D. Singh, K. Tubesing, et al. Cutaneous photoprotection from ultraviolet injury by green tea polyphenols. *Journal of the American Academy of Dermatology.* 2001; 44 (3): 425–432.

Foster, S., J. A. Duke. *Eastern/Central Medicinal Plants.* New York: Houghton Mifflin, 1990.

Fujita, H., T. Yamagami. Antihypercholesterolemic effect of Chinese black tea extract in human subjects with borderline hypercholesterolemia. *Nutr Res.* 2008; 28 (7): 450–456.

Fukino, Y., A. Ikeda, K. Maruyama, N. Aoki, T. Okubo, H. Iso. Randomized controlled trial for an effect of green tea-extract powder supplementation on glucose abnormalities. *Eur J Clin Nutr.* 2007; Epub ahead of print.

Fukuda, I., I. Sakane, Y. Yabushita, et al. Black tea theaflavins suppress dioxin-induced transformation of the aryl hydrocarbon receptor. *Biosci Biotechnol Biochem.* 2005; 69: 883–890.

Geleijnse, J. M., L. J. Launer, A. Hofman, et al. Tea flavonoids may protect against hardening of the arteries: the Rotterdam Study. *Arch Intern Med.* 1999; 159: 2170–2174.

Geleijnse, J. M., J. C. Witteman, L. J. Launer, et al. Tea and coronary heart disease: protection through estrogen-like activity? *Arch Intern Med.* 2000; 160: 3328–3329.

Graham, H.N. Green tea composition, consumption, and polyphenol chemistry. *Prev Med.* 1992; 21 (3): 334–350.

Gross, G., K. G. Meyer, H. Pres, C. Thielert, H. Tawfik, A. Mescheder. A randomized, double-blind, four-arm parallel-group, placebo-controlled Phase II/III study to investigate the clinical efficacy of two galenic formulations of Polyphenon(R) E in the treatment of external genital warts. *J Eur Acad Dermatol Venereol.* 2007; 21 (10): 1404–1412.

Hakim, I. A., R. B. Harris, S. Brown, et al. Effect of increased tea consumption on oxidative DNA damage among smokers: A randomized controlled study. *Journal of Nutrition.* 2003; 133 (10): 3303S–3309S.

Haller, C. A., N. L. Benowitz, P. Jacob III. Hemodynamic effects of ephedra-free weight-loss supplements in humans. *Am J Med.* 2005; 118: 998–1003.

Hartman, T. J., J. A. Tangrea, P. Pietinen, et al. Tea and coffee consumption and risk of colon and rectal cancer in middle-aged Finnish men. *Nutr Cancer.* 1998; 31: 41–48.

Heck, A. M., B. A. DeWitt, A. L. Lukes. Potential interactions between alternative therapies and warfarin, review. *Am J Health Syst Pharm.* 2000 Jul 1; 57 (13): 1221–1227.

Hegarty, V. M., H. M. May, K. Khaw. Tea drinking and bone mineral density in older women. *Am J Clin Nutr.* 2000; 7 1: 1003–1007.

Henning, S. M., Y. Niu, N. H. Lee, et al. Bioavailability and antioxidant activity of tea flavanols after consumption of green tea, black tea, or a green tea extract supplement. *J. Clin. Nutr.* 2004; 80 (6): 1558–1564.

Hernandez-Avila, M., G. A. Colditz, M. J. Stampfer, B. Rosner, F. E. Speizer, W. C. Willett. Caffeine, moderate alcohol intake, and risk of fractures of the hip and forearm in middle-aged women. *Am J Clin Nutr.* 1991; 54 (1): 157–163.

Hernandez-Avila, M., M. J. Stampfer, V. A. Ravnikar, et al. Caffeine and other predictors of bone density among pre- and perimenopausal women. *Epidemiology.* 1993 ;4 (2): 128–134.

Higdon, J. V., B. Frei. Coffee and health: A review of recent human research. *Critical Reviews in Food Science and Nutrition.* 2006; 46 (2): 101–123.

————. Tea catechins and polyphenols: health effects, metabolism, and antioxidant functions. *Crit Rev Food Sci Nutr.* 2003; 43 (1): 89–143.

Hindmarch, I., P. T. Quinlan, K. L. Moore, C. Parkin. The effects of black tea and other beverages on aspects of cognition and psychomotor performance. *Psychopharmacol.* 1998; 139: 230–238.

Hirasawa, M., K. Takada, S. Otake. Inhibition of acid production in dental plaque bacteria by green tea catechins. *Caries Res.* 2006; 40 (3): 265–270.

Hodgson, J. M., I. B. Puddey, V. Burke, et al. Effects on blood pressure of drinking green and black tea. *J Hypertens.* 1999; 17: 457–463.

Hodgson, J. M., I. B. Puddey, K. D. Croft, et al. Acute effects of ingestion of black and green tea on lipoprotein oxidation. *Am J Clin Nutr.* 2000; 71: 1103–1107.

Hoshiyama, Y., T. Kawaguchi, Y. Miura, et al. A nested case-control study of stomach cancer in relation to green tea consumption in Japan. *Br J Cancer.* 2004; 90 (1): 135–138.

————. Green tea and stomach cancer—a short review of prospective studies. *J Epidemiol.* 2005; 15 Suppl 2: S109–112.

Hou, Z., J. D. Lambert, K. V. Chin, C. S. Yang. Effects of tea polyphenols on signal transduction pathways related to cancer chemoprevention. *Mutat Res.* 2004; 555 (1–2): 3–19.

Howell, L.L., V. L. Coffin, R. D. Spealman. Behavioral and physiological effects of xanthines in nonhuman primates. *Psychopharmacology.* (Berl) 1997; 129: 1–14.

Hsu, C.H., Y. L. Liao, S. C. Lin, T. H. Tsai, C. J. Huang, P. Chou. Does supplementation with green tea extract improve insulin resistance in obese type 2 diabetics? A randomized, double-blind, and placebo-controlled clinical trial. *Altern Med Rev.* 2011 Jun; 16 (2): 157–163.

Infante, S., M. L. Baeza, M. Calvo, et al. Anaphylaxis due to caffeine. *Allergy.* 2003; 58: 681–682.

Inoue, M., K. Tajima, K. Hirose, et al. Tea and coffee consumption and the risk of digestive tract cancers: data from a comparative case-referent study in Japan. *Cancer Causes Control.* 1998; 9: 209–216.

Inoue, M., K. Tajima, M. Mizutani, et al. Regular consumption of green tea and the risk of breast cancer recurrence: follow-up study from the Hospital-based Epidemiologic Research Program at Aichi Cancer Center (HERPACC), Japan. *Cancer Lett.* 2001; 167(2): 175–182.

Iso, H., C. Date, K. Wakai, et al. JACC Study Group. The relationship between green tea and total caffeine intake and risk for self-reported type 2 diabetes among Japanese adults. *Ann Intern Med.* 2006; 144: 554–562.

Jatoi, A., N. Ellison, P. A. Burch, et al. A phase II trial of green tea in the treatment of patients with androgen independent metastatic prostate carcinoma. *Cancer.* 2003; 97 (6): 1442–1446.

Jian, L., A. H. Lee, C. W. Binns. Tea and lycopene protect against prostate cancer. *Asian Pacific Journal of Clinical Nutrition.* 2007; 16 (Suppl 1): 453–457.

Jian, L., L. P. Xie, A. H. Lee, C. W. Binns. Protective effect of green tea against prostate cancer: a case-control study in southeast China. *Int J Cancer.* Jan 1, 2004; 108 (1): 130–135.

Jin, X., R. H. Zheng, Y. M. Li. Green tea consumption and liver disease: a systematic review. *Liver Int.* 2008; 28 (7): 990–996.

Johnell O., B. Gullberg, J. A. Kanis, et al. Risk factors for hip fracture in European women: the MEDOS Study. Mediterranean Osteoporosis Study. *J Bone Miner Res.* 1995; 10 (11): 1802–1815.

Kanis, J., O. Johnell, B. Gullberg, et al. Risk factors for hip fracture in men from southern Europe: the MEDOS study. Mediterranean Osteoporosis Study. *Osteoporos Int.* 1999; 9: 45–54.

Katiyar, S. K., N. Ahmad, H. Mukhtar. Green tea and skin. *Arch Dermatol.* 2000; 136 (8): 989–994.

Kato, A., Y. Minoshima, J. Yamamoto, I. Adachi, A. A. Watson, R. J. Nash. Protective effects of dietary chamomile tea on diabetic complications. *J Agric Food Chem.* 2008; 56 (17): 8206–8211.

Kimura, K., M. Ozeki, L. R. Juneja, H. Ohira. L-Theanine reduces psychological and physiological stress responses. *Biol Psychol.* 2007; 74 (1): 39–45.

Koizumi, Y., Y. Tsubono, N. Nakaya, et al. No association between green tea and the risk of gastric cancer: pooled analysis of two prospective studies in Japan. *Cancer Epidemiol Biomarkers Prev.* 2003; 12 (5): 472–473.

Komatsu, T., M. Nakamori, K. Komatsu, et al. Oolong tea increases energy metabolism in Japanese females. *J Med Invest.* 2003; 50 (3–4): 170–175.

Koo, S. I., S. K. Noh. Green tea as inhibitor of the intestinal absorption of lipids: potential mechanism for its lipid-lowering effect. *J Nutr Biochem.* 2007; 18 (3): 179–83.

Kovacs, E. M., M. P. Lejeune, I. Nijs, M. S. Westerterp-Plantenga. Effects of green tea on weight maintenance after body-weight loss. *Br J Nutr.* Mar 1, 2004; 91 (3): 431–437.

Kreuz, S., E. Joubert, K. H. Waldemann, W. Ternes. Aspalathin, a flavonoid in aspalathus linearis (rooibos) is absorbed by pig intenstine as C-glycoside. *Nutr. Res.,* 2008; Oct 28 (10): 651–658.

Kundu, T., S. Dey, M. Roy, et al. Induction of apoptosis in human leukemia cells by black tea and its polyphenol theaflavin. *Cancer Lett.* 2005; 230: 111–121.

Kurahashi ,N., S. Sasazuki, M. Iwasaki, M. Inoue, S. Tsugane. Green tea consumption and prostate cancer risk in Japanese men: A prospective study. *American Journal of Epidemiology.* 2008; 167 (1): 71–77.

Kuriyama, S., T. Shimazu, K. Ohmori, N. Kikuchi, N. Nakaya, Y. Nishino, Y. Tsubono, I. Tsuji. Green tea consumption and mortality due to cardiovascular disease, cancer and all causes in Japan: the Ohsaki study. *JAMA.* 2006; 296 (10): 1255–1265.

Lanio, C. Hibiscus tea may cut blood pressure. www
.webmd.com/heart/news/20081110/hibiscus
-tea-may-cut-blood-pressure.

Lambert, J. D., C. S. Yang. Mechanisms of cancer
prevention by tea constituents. *Journal of Nutrition.*
2003; 133 (10): 3262S–3267S.

Larsson, S. C., A. Wolk. Tea consumption and ovarian
cancer risk in a population-based cohort. *Arch
Intern Med.* 2005; 165: 2683–2686.

Lee W., W. K. Min, S. Chun, Y. W. Lee, H. Park, D.
H. Lee, Y. K. Lee, J. E. Son. Long-term effects of
green tea ingestion on atherosclerotic biological
markers in smokers. *Clin Biochem.* Jan 1, 2005; 38
(1): 84–87.

Leenen, R., A. J. Roodenburg, L. B. Tijburg, et al. A
single dose of tea with or without milk increases
plasma antioxidant activity in humans. *Eur J Clin
Nutr.* 2000; 54: 87–92.

Leung, L. K., Y. Su, R. Chen, et al. Theaflavins in black
tea and catechins in green tea are equally effective
antioxidants. *J Nutr.* 2001; 131: 2248–2251.

Li, N., Sun, Z., Han, C., J. Chen. The chemopreventive
effects of tea on human oral precancerous mucosa
lesions. *Proceedings from the Society of Experimental
Biology and Medicine.* 1999; 220 (4): 218–224.

Li, Q., M. Kakizaki, S. Kuriyama, et al. Green tea consumption and lung cancer risk: The Ohsaki study. *British Journal of Cancer.* 2008; 99 (7): 1179–1184.

Linke, H. A., R. Z. LeGeros. Black tea extract and dental caries formation in hamsters. *Int J Food Sci Nutr.* 2003; 54 (1): 89–95.

Liu, S., H. Lu, Q. Zhao, et al. Theaflavin derivatives in black tea and catechin derivatives in green tea inhibit HIV-1 entry by targeting gp41. *Biochim Biophys Acta.* 2005;1 723: 270–281.

Lorenz, M., N. Jochmann, A. von Krosigk, et al. Addition of milk prevents vascular protective effects of tea. *Eur Heart J.* 2007; 28: 219–223.

Low Dog, T., D. Riley, T. Carter. Traditional and alternative therapies for breast cancer. *Alt Ther.* 2001; 7 (3): 36–47.

Lu, Y. P., Lou, Y. R., Y. Lin, et al. Inhibitory effects of orally administered green tea, black tea, and caffeine on skin carcinogenesis in mice previously treated with ultraviolet B light (high-risk mice): relationship to decreased tissue fat. *Cancer Res.* 2001; 61 (13): 5002–5009.

Lu, Q. *Clinical Cancer Research.* Feb. 15, 2005; vol 11: 1–9.

Lu, T., H. Sheng, J. Wu, et al. Cinnamon reduces hemoglobin A1C and blood glucose. *Nutr. Res.* June 2012; 32 (6): 408–412.

Luo, H., L. Tang, M. Tang, et al. Phase IIa chemo-prevention trial of green tea polyphenols in high-risk individuals of liver cancer: Modulation of urinary excretion of green tea polyphenols and 8-hydroxydeoxyguanosine. *Carcinogenesis* 2006; 27 (2): 262–268.

Manach, C., A. Scalbert, C. Morand, C, Remesy, L. Jimenez. Polyphenols: food sources and bioavailability. *Am J Clin Nutr.* 2004; 79 (5): 727–747.

Maron, D.J., G. P. Lu, N. S. Cai, et al. Cholesterol-lowering effect of a theaflavin-enriched green tea extract: a randomized controlled trial. *Arch Intern Med* 2003; 163: 1448–1453.

Massey, L.K., H. Roman-Smith, R. A. Sutton. Effect of dietary oxalate and calcium on urinary oxalate and risk of formation of calcium oxalate kidney stones. *J Am Diet Assoc.* 1993; 93 (8): 901–906.

Massey, L.K., S. J. Whiting. Caffeine, urinary calcium, calcium metabolism and bone. *J Nutr* 1993; 123: 1611–1614.

Massey, L.K. Tea oxalate. *Nutr Rev.* 2000; 58 (3 pt 1): 88–89.

Matsumoto, M., T. Minami, H. Sasaki, S. Sobue, S. Hamada, T. Ooshima. Inhibitory effects of oolong tea extract on caries-inducing properties of mutans streptococci. *Caries Res.* 1999; 33 (6): 441–445.

McKay, D.L. Hibiscus tea can lower hypertension. Paper presented at the Am Heart Assoc conference, Nov 8–12, 2008.

McKenna, D.J., K. Hughes, K. Jones. Green tea monograph. *Alt Ther.* 2000; 6 (3): 61–84.

Michels, K.B., L. Holmberg, L. Bergkvist, A. Wolk. Coffee, tea, and caffeine consumption and breast cancer incidence in a cohort of Swedish women. *Ann Epidimiol,* 2002 Jan; 12 (1): 21–26.

Migliardi, J.R., J.J. Armellino, M. Friedman, et al. Caffeine as an analgesic adjuvant in tension headache. *Clin Pharmacol Ther* 1994; 56: 576–586.

Miura, Y., T. Chiba, I. Tomita, et al. Tea catechins prevent the development of hardening of the arteries in apoprotein E-deficient mice. *J Nutr.* 2001; 131 (1): 27–32.

Mukhtar, H., N. Ahmad. Tea polyphenols: Prevention of cancer and optimizing health. *American Journal of Clinical Nutrition* 2000; 71 (6 Suppl): 1698S–1702S.

Nagao, T., T. Hase, I. Tokimitsu. A green tea extract high in catechins reduces body fat and cardiovascular risks in humans. *Obesity* (Silver Spring). 2007; 15 (6):1473–1483.

Nagao, T., Y. Komine, S. Soga, et al. Ingestion of a tea rich in catechins leads to a reduction in body fat and malondialdehyde-modified LDL in men. *Am J Clin Nutr.* 2005; 81(1): 122–129.

Nagao, T. *Obesity*, June 2007; vol 15: 1473–1483.

Nascimento, G. G. F., J. Locatelli, P. C. Freitas, G. L. Silva. Antibacterial activity of plant extracts and phytochemicals on antibiotic-resistant bacteria. *Braz. J. Microbiol,* 2000; 31 (4): 247–256.

Nawrot, P., S. Jordan, J. Eastwood, et al. Effects of caffeine on human health. *Food Addit Contam* 2003; 20: 1–30.

Nurminen, M.L., L. Niittynen, R. Korpela, H. Vapaatalo. Coffee, caffeine and blood pressure: a critical review. *Eur J Clin Nutr* 1999; 53: 831–839.

Peters, U., C. Poole, L. Arab. Does tea affect cardiovascular disease? A meta-analysis. *Am J Epidemiol* 2001; 154: 495–503.

Peterson, J., J. Dwyer, P. Jacques, et al. Tea variety and brewing techniques influence flavonoid content of black tea. *Journal of Food Composition and Analysis* 2004; 17 (3–4): 397–405.

Pianetti, S., S. Guo, K. T. Kavanagh, G. E. Sonenshein. Green tea polyphenol epigallocatechin-3 gallate inhibits Her-2/neu signaling, proliferation, and transformed phenotype of breast cancer cells. *Cancer Res.* 2002; 62 (3): 652–655.

Pisters, K. M., R. A. Newman, B. Coldman, et al. Phase I trial of oral green tea extract in adult patients with solid tumors. *J Clin Oncol.* 2001; 19 (6): 1830–1838.

Pollock, B.G., M. Wylie, J. A. Stack, et al. Inhibition of caffeine metabolism by estrogen replacement therapy in postmenopausal women. *J Clin Pharmacol* 1999; 39: 936–940.

Rakic V., L. J. Beilin, V. Burke. Effect of coffee and tea drinking on postprandial hypotension in older men and women. *Clin Exp Pharmacol Physiol* 1996; 23: 559–563.

Rasheed, A., M. Haider. Antibacterial activity of Camellia sinensis extracts against dental caries. *Arch Pharm Res.* 1998; 21 (3): 348–352.

Reto, M., M. E. Figueira, H. M. Filipe, C. M. Almeida. Chemical composition of green tea (*Camellia sinensis*) infusions commercialized in Portugal. *Plant Foods for Human Nutrition* 2007; 62 (4): 139–144.

Robinson, L.E., S. Savani, D. S. Battram, et al. Caffeine ingestion before an oral glucose tolerance test impairs blood glucose management in men with type 2 diabetes. *J Nutr* 2004; 134: 2528–2533.

Ross, G.W., R. D. Abbott, H. Petrovitch, et al. Association of coffee and caffeine intake with the risk of parkinson disease. *JAMA* 2000; 283: 2674–2679.

Rowe, C.A., M. P. Nantz, J. F. Bukowski, S. S. Percival. Specific formulation of Camellia sinensis prevents cold and flu symptoms and enhances gammadelta T cell function: a randomized, double-blind, placebo-controlled study. *J Am Coll Nutr.* 2007; 26 (5): 445–452.

Rumpler, W., J. Seale, B. Clevidence, et al. Oolong tea increases metabolic rate and fat oxidation in men. *J Nutr.* 2001; 131 (11): 2848–2852.

Ryu OH, Lee J, Lee KW, et al. Effects of green tea consumption on inflammation, insulin resistance and pulse wave velocity in type 2 diabetes patients. *Diabetes Res Clin Pract.* 2006; 71 (3): 356–358.

Sandeep, T, L. Licorice and Cognitive Function. *Proceedings of the National Academy of Sciences*, March 29, 2004, vol 101.

Sano ,T., M. Sasako. Green tea and gastric cancer. *N Engl J Med.* 2001; 344 (9): 675–676.

Santana-Rios G., G. A. Orner, A. Amantana, C. Provost, S. Y. Wu, R. H. Dashwood. Potent antimutagenic activity of white tea in comparison with green tea in the Salmonella assay. *Mutat Res.* 2001; 495 (1–2): 61–74.

Santana-Rios, G., G. A. Orner, M. Xu, M. Izquierdo-Pulido, R. H. Dashwood. Inhibition by white tea of 2-amino-1-methyl-6-phenylimidazo 4,5-b pyridine-induced colonic aberrant crypts in the F344 rat. *Nutrition and Cancer* 2001; 41 (1 and 2): 98–103.

Sasazuki, S., H. Kodama, K. Yoshimasu, et al. Relation between green tea consumption and the severity of coronary hardening of the arteries among Japanese men and women. *Ann Epidemiol.* 2000; 10: 401–408.

Schabath, M. B., L. M. Hernandez, X. Wu, et al. Dietary phytoestrogens and lung cancer risk. *JAMA* 2005; 294: 1493–1504.

Setiawan, V. W., Z. F. Zhang, G. P. Yu, et al. Protective effect of green tea on the risks of chronic gastritis and stomach cancer. *Int J Cancer.* 2001; 92(4): 600–604.

Shahrzad, S., K. Aoyagi, A. Winter, et al. Pharmacokinetics of gallic acid and its relative bioavailability from tea in healthy humans. *J Nutr* 2001; 131: 1207–1210.

Shankar, S., S. Ganapathy, S. R. Hingorani, R. K. Srivastava. EGCG inhibits growth, invasion, angiogenesis and metastasis of pancreatic cancer. *Front Biosci.* 2008; 13: 440–452.

Sherman, G. "Tea's health benefits boost its popularity." April 1, 2003. http://www.washingtonpost.com/national/health-science/teas-health-benefits-boost-its-popularity/2013/04/01/be818cfe-6ef5-11e2-aa58-243de81040ba_story.html.

Silvera, S. A., M. Jain, G. R. Howe, A. B. Miller, T. E. Rohan. Intake of coffee and tea and risk of ovarian cancer: A prospective cohort study. *Nutrition and Cancer* 2007; 58 (1): 22–27.

Steele, V. E., G. J. Kelloff, D. Balentine, et al. Comparative chemopreventive mechanisms of green tea, black tea and selected polyphenol extracts measured by in vitro bioassays. *Carcinogenesis* 2000; 21 (1): 63–67.

Steptoe, A., E. L. Gibson, R. Vuonovirta, M. Hamer, J. Wardle, J. A. Rycroft, J. F. Martin, J. D. Erusalimsky. The effects of chronic tea intake on platelet activation and inflammation: a double-blind placebo controlled trial. *Hardening of the Arteries.* 2007; 193 (2): 277–282.

Su, L. J., L. Arab. Tea consumption and the reduced risk of colon cancer —results from a national prospective cohort study. *Public Health Nutr* 2002; 5: 419–425.

Sun, C.L., J. M. Yuan, W. P. Koh,H. P. Lee, M. C. Yu. Green tea and black tea consumption in relation to colorectal cancer risk: The Singapore Chinese Health Study. *Carcinogenesis* 2007; 28 (10): 2143–2148.

Suzuki, Y., Y. Tsubono, N. Nakaya, Y. Suzuki,Y. Koizumi, I. Tsuji. Green tea and the risk of breast cancer: pooled analysis of two prospective studies in Japan. *Br J Cancer.* Apr 5, 2004; 90 (7): 1361–1363.

Tajima, K., S. Tominaga. Dietary habits and gastro-intestinal cancers: a comparative case-control study of stomach and large intestinal cancers in Nagoya, Japan. *Jpn J Cancer Res* 1985; 76: 705–16.

Tang, N., Y. Wu, B. Zhou, B. Wang, R. Yu. Green tea, black tea consumption and risk of lung cancer: A meta-analysis. *Lung Cancer* 2009; 65 (3): 274–283.

Taubert, D., R. Roesen, E. Schomig. Effect of cocoa and tea intake on blood pressure: a meta-analysis. *Arch Intern Med* 2007; 167: 626–634.

Tavani, A., C. L. Vecchia. Coffee, decaffeinated coffee, tea and cancer of the colon and rectum: a review of epidemiological studies, 1990-2003. *Cancer Causes Control.* 2004; 15 (8): 743–757.

Terry, P., A. Wolk. Tea consumption and the risk of colorectal cancer in Sweden. *Nutr Cancer* 2001; 39: 176–179.

Thatte, U., S. Bagadey, S. Dahanukar. Modulation of programmed cell death by medicinal plants. Review . *Cell Mol Biol.* 2000; 46 (1): 199–214.

Thavanesan, N. The putative effects of green tea on body fat: an evaluation of the evidence and a review of the potential mechanisms. *Br J Nutr.* 2011 Aug 3: 1–13.

Trevisanato, S. I., Y. I. Kim. Tea and health. *Nutr Rev.* 2000; 58 (1): 1–10.

Tsubono, Y., Y. Nishino, S. Komatsu, et al. Green tea and the risk of gastric cancer in Japan. *N Engl J Med.* 2001; 344 (9): 632–636.

Vinson, J.A., K. Teufel, N. Wu. Green and black teas inhibit hardening of the arteries by lipid, antioxidant, and fibrinolytic mechanisms. *J Agric Food Chem* 2004; 52: 3661–3665.

Wang, L., I. M. Lee, S. M. Zhang, et al. Dietary intake of selected flavonols, flavones, and flavonoid-rich foods and risk of cancer in middle-aged and older women. *American Journal of Clinical Nutrition* 2009; 89 (3): 905–912.

Wang, L. D., Q. Zhou, C. W. Feng, et al. Intervention and follow-up on human esophageal precancerous lesions in Henan, northern China, a high-incidence area for esophageal cancer. *Gan To Kagaku Ryoho* 2002; 29 (suppl 1): 159–172.

Wargovich, M.J., C. Woods, D. M. Hollis, M. E. Zander. Herbals, cancer prevention and health. Review .*J Nutr.* 2001; 131 (11 suppl): 3034S–3036S.

Watson, J. M., R. S. Sherwin, I. J. Deary, et al. Dissociation of augmented physiological, hormonal and cognitive responses to hypoglycaemia with sustained caffeine use. *Clin Sci* (Lond) 2003; 104: 447–454.

Way, T. D., H. H. Lee, M. C. Kao, J. K. Lin. Black tea polyphenol theaflavins inhibit aromatase activity and attenuate tamoxifen resistance in HER2/ neu-transfected human breast cancer cells through tyrosine kinase suppression. *European Journal of Cancer,* 2004; 40: 2165–2174.

Westerterp-Plantenga M.S., M. P. Lejeune, E. M. Kovacs. Body weight and weight maintenance in relation to habitual caffeine intake and green tea. *Obes Res* Jul 2005; 13 (7): 1195–1204.

Wilbert, C. "Prevent diabetic ills with chamomile tea?" www.webmd.com/diabetes/news/20080911 /prevent-diabetic-ills-with-chamomile-tea

Winkelmayer, W. C., M. J. Stampfer, W. C. Willett, G. C. Curhan. Habitual caffeine intake and the risk of hypertension in women. *JAMA* 2005; 294: 2330–2335.

Wu, A.H., I. M. Butler. Green tea and breast cancer. *Mol Nutr Food Res.* 2011 Jun; 55 (6): 921–930.

Wu, A.H., C. C. Tseng, D. Van Den Berg, M. C. Yu. Tea intake, COMT genotype, and breast cancer in Asian-American women. *Cancer Res.* 2003 ;63 (21): 7526–7529.

Wu, C.H., Y.C. Yang, W. J. Yao, F. H. Lu, J.S. Wu, C. J. Chang. Epidemiological evidence of increased bone mineral density in habitual tea drinkers. *Arch Intern Med.* 2002; 162 (9): 1001–1006.

Yang C.S., P. Maliakal, X. Meng. Inhibition of carcinogenesis by tea. *Annual Review of Pharmacology and Toxicology* 2002; 42: 25–54.

Yang G., X. O. Shu, H. Li, W. H. Chow, B. T. Ji, X. Zhang, Y. T. Gao, W. Zheng. Prospective cohort study of green tea consumption and colorectal cancer risk in women. *Cancer Epidemiol Biomarkers Prev.* 2007; 16(6): 1219–1223.

Yang G., W. Zheng, Y. B. Xiang, J. Gao, H. L. Li, X. Zhang, Y. T. Gao, X. O. Shu. Green tea consumption and colorectal cancer risk: a report from the Shanghai Men's Health Study. *Carcinogenesis.* 2011 Sep 8. Epub ahead of print.

Yuan J.M. Green tea and prevention of esophageal and lung cancers. *Mol Nutr Food Res.* 2011 Jun; 55 (6): 886–904.

Zaveri N.T. Green tea and its polyphenolic catechins: Medicinal uses in cancer and noncancer applications. *Life Sciences* 2006; 78 (18): 2073–2080.

Zhang M.,C. W. Binns, A. H. Lee. Tea consumption and ovarian cancer risk: a case-control study in China. *Cancer Epidemiol Biomarkers Prev* 2002; 11: 713–718.

Zhang M., C. D. Holman, J. P. Huang, X. Xie. Green tea and the prevention of breast cancer: A case-control study in Southeast China. *Carcinogenesis* 2007; 28 (5): 1074–1078.

Zhang M., A. H. Lee, C. W. Binns, X. Xie. Green tea consumption enhances survival of epithelial ovarian cancer. *Int J Cancer* 2004, Nov 10; 112 (3): 465–469.

Zheng, J., B. Yang, T. Huang, Y. Yu, J. Yang, D. Li. Green tea and black tea consumption and prostate cancer risk: an exploratory meta-analysis of observational studies. *Nutr Cancer.* 2011;63 (5): 663–672. Epub 2011 Jun 11.

Zhou B., L. Yang, L. Wang, et al. The association of tea consumption with ovarian cancer risk: A metaanalysis. *American Journal of Obstetrics and Gynecology* 2007; 197 (6): 594.e1–e6.

Zijp I.M., O. Korver, L.B. Tijburg. Effect of tea and other dietary factors on iron absorption. *Crit Rev Food Sci Nutr* 2000; 40: 371–398.

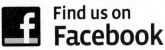 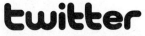
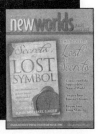

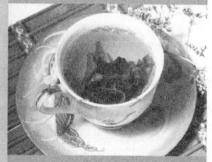

Tea Leaf
Reading

For Beginners

Your Fortune in a Tea Cup

CAROLINE DOW

Tea Leaf Reading for Beginners
Your Fortune in a Tea Cup
CAROLINE DOW

More people than ever are discovering the restorative benefits of tea and the life-enriching divinatory practice of tea-leaf reading. In answer to the surging popularity of this healthful and mystical beverage, *Tea Leaf Reading for Beginners* teaches readers how to read and interpret tea-leaves in six simple steps.

This complete guidebook explores the origins of tea and tea-leaf reading, ways of giving readings, divination ethics, tea's medicinal uses, herbal infusion preparation, and how to host a tea party. For quick and easy interpretation, hundreds of symbols and their meanings are included, organized by theme—animals, sun signs, plants, shapes, and many others.

978-0-7387-2329-7, 312 pp., 5³⁄₁₆ x 8   **$15.95**

HOMEOPATHY
An A to Z Home Handbook

Alan V.
Schmukler

Homeopathy
An A to Z Home Handbook
ALAN V. SCHMUKLER

Effective, safe, affordable, and free of chemical side effects—the benefits of homeopathy are endless! Already established in the national health care systems of England, France, Germany, and the Netherlands, homeopathic treatments are used by over 500 million people worldwide. Alan Schmukler's *Homeopathy* discusses the history and science of this alternative medicine and provides a comprehensive list of proven remedies—safe for people and animals.

Packed with homeopathic treatments for arthritis, colds, food poisoning, insomnia, Lyme disease, morning sickness, wounds, and a host of other ailments and injuries, this handy reference guide also includes information on homeopathic immunization and first aid. Schmukler gives helpful instructions for matching remedies with symptoms, ingesting them correctly, making remedies at home, and stretching your supply.

978-0-7387-0873-7, 360 pp., 6 x 9   **$17.95**

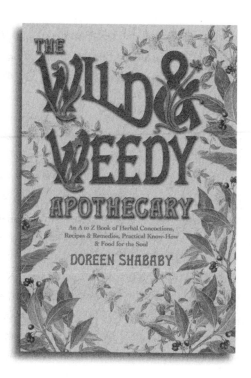

THE WILD & WEEDY APOTHECARY

An A to Z Book of Herbal Concoctions,
Recipes & Remedies, Practical Know-How
& Food for the Soul

DOREEN SHABABY

The Wild & Weedy Apothecary
An A to Z Book of Herbal Concoctions, Recipes &
Remedies, Practical Know-How & Food for the Soul
DOREEN SHABABY

Step off the beaten path and into nature's wild and weedy apothecary. In this warm and friendly guide, herbalist Doreen Shababy shares her deep, abiding love for the earth and its gifts. She invites readers to be playful and adventurous as they learn how to use herbs to make a soothing salve, fragrant tea, vibrant salads, and other dishes to delight the palate as well as the eye.

This extensive collection of herbal remedies, folk and food wisdom, and eclectic recipes from around the world represents a lifetime of the author's work in the forest, field, and kitchen. Organized in an easy and fun A to Z format, Shababy's extensive knowledge of the subject and unique collection of wit and wisdom will speak to beginners and herb enthusiasts alike.

978-0-7387-1907-8, 384 pp., 6 x 9   **$17.95**
